St Tiggywinkles
Wildcare Handbook

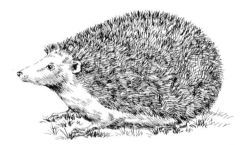

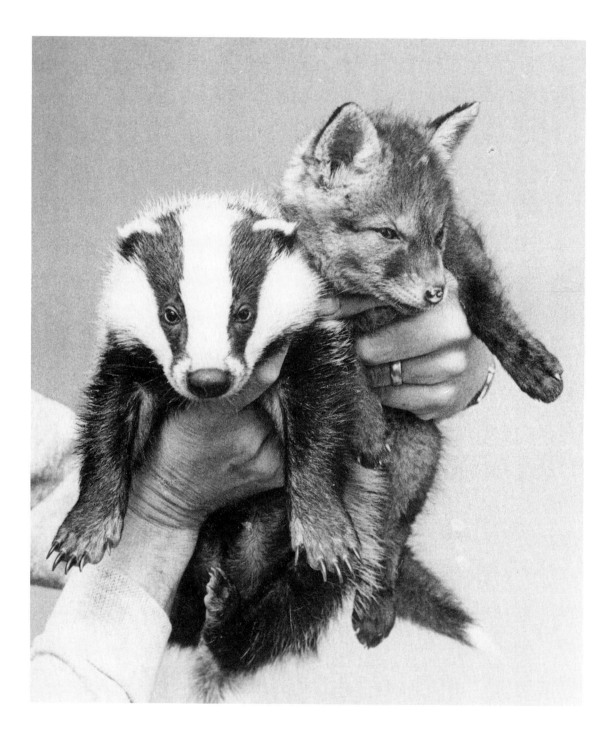

St Tiggywinkles
Wildcare Handbook

First Aid & Care for Wildlife

Les Stocker

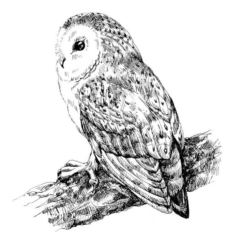

Chatto & Windus

LONDON

By the same author:
The Complete Hedgehog
Something In A Cardboard Box
The Hedgehog And Friends
The Complete Garden Bird

Published in 1992 by
Chatto & Windus Ltd
20 Vauxhall Bridge Road
London SW1V 2SA

A CIP catalogue record for this book is available from the
British Library

ISBN 0 7011 3775 4

Line illustrations by Stevie Wilkinson
Designed by Behram Kapadia
Photoset by Rowland Phototypesetting Ltd,
Bury St Edmunds, Suffolk
Printed in Great Britain by Butler and Tanner Ltd
Frome, Somerset

Contents

BIRD AND MAMMAL AID CHARTS

Introduction

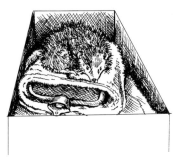

I find it very heartening that, in the 1990s the plight of the wildlife casualty is being taken up by increasing numbers of good people. Over the past fifteen years I have encountered thousands of wild animals and birds and they have all shown such a will to survive that I have felt it my duty and privilege to help, and to help others help them.

A decade and a half ago the Wildlife Hospital Trust, affectionately known as St Tiggywinkles, was set up by myself, my wife Sue and son Colin, to offer help to all those sick or injured wild animals and birds which were being ignored or killed. The commonly used phrase at the time was 'it's only nature' or 'put it out of its misery'.

My experiences over those years have shown me that 95% of all wildlife casualties are injured as a result of their encounters with man and his artificial environment. We owe it to these victims to try to make amends for some of the hazards we have put in their way.

Nature has little part in this conflict – you have only to look at the small proportion of casualties we receive whose injuries come from natural rather than man-made causes. To my mind, that statement 'put it out of its misery' is too often an abdication of responsibility and avoidance of the cost involved in treating an injured animal (a treated animal may need months to recuperate and hardly any vets or welfare centres have facilities to keep live animals for longer than a day or two).

And just what *is* misery? Every animal I see wants to live. It does not think of its pain as misery. But then, given the right care and treatment, that pain or suffering can be relieved, it is soon past and the animal thrives, raring to go. It won't thank you, it won't even remember your care, but it will be fit and free again.

Over the years we have had to learn techniques to use in caring for Britain's wildlife. There was no teaching available to us, very little literature and hardly anyone around with experience to pass on. We have had to improvise, adapt, innovate, fail and succeed with all manner of injuries and infected wounds, the kind not normally seen in dogs and cats or at a vet's surgery or animal welfare clinic. But succeed we have and most of our casualties have now been returned to their wild existence, where they flourish.

This book is the culmination of all our experiences. It is not a veterinary manual, rather it attempts to show you how *you* can help wild animals and birds at a basic level. Only when the treatments require the sophisticated techniques of a veterinary surgeon do I recommend that you approach one, and even then I point out that some vets will work on wildlife while others flatly refuse. But you are paying the bill and you have a right to demand the best for your animal. It has as much right to life and the proper treatment as a dog or cat, so insist on it.

Conservative estimates in this country give the number of wild creatures that don't die instantly from their injuries to be in excess of five million every year. I would love to be able to help each and every one of them but that is simply not possible. I have therefore written this book to encourage and inform others; we have also just built the world's first wildlife teaching hospital, where we can not only treat casualties but where others – laymen, vets and nurses – can come on courses to learn about the intricacies of wild animals and their treatment. Those people will also, I hope, come up with their own innovations in wildlife treatment and care. Then more people around Britain can take in wildlife casualties, and together we may be able to make a dent in that five million, as well as relieving a lot of pain and saving many needlessly wasted lives.

This handbook has been laid out for easy reference but a word of warning: in my experience an obvious problem affecting a casualty could be masking all manner of other ailments. For this reason I would recommend reading the book from cover to cover before you even look at your first animal. Then, and only then, can you use it efficiently as a quick reference guide, since you will be aware that there might be some other problem you have read about.

Lastly, although the majority of vets do not deal regularly with

Suggested first-aid kit: Birds and Mammals (see Appendices I, II for suppliers)

Stout cardboard box with lid and airholes punched around the bottom
Heated cage, mat or ceramic heater
Old towel (clean but with no holes or loose threads)
2.5cm zinc oxide plaster
Non-adhesive dressing – Melolin
Non-adhesive cohesive bandage
Lacri-Lube ocular lubricant (Allergan)
Savlon or Hibiscrub
Surgical spirit
Cotton wool
Cotton buds
Surgical gauze
Bamboo cane or strips of wood for leg splints
Chloramphenicol eye ointment (POM★)
Columbo-clips
Artery forceps
Spreull's needles, 2, 5 & 10ml syringes
Sterile needle (to lance abscesses)
Leather gloves (for handling hedgehogs and birds of prey)
Small scissors
Dexamethasone (POM★)
Caustic pencil
Potassium permanganate
Lectade
Liquid paraffin
Various low-sided food or water containers (and budgerigar's gravity-fed 'water fountain' if possible)

Mammals only

Fluid administration kit (see Ch. 6, p. 136)
Battle fly and maggot paste
Curved scissors
Hydrogen peroxide solution 20vols (6%)
5cm cotton bandage
Plastic leg splints

★POM means Prescription-Only Medicine. That is, it can only be prescribed by a vet.

wildlife casualties, it is essential that anyone contemplating treating a patient with a serious injury should work with a sympathetic veterinary surgeon. We at St Tiggywinkles have always worked closely with vets and have now produced a Code of Practice to establish who can do what and when.

THE MOST IMPORTANT THING TO REMEMBER IS THAT THE ANIMAL'S WELFARE IS PARAMOUNT AND THAT IT WANTS TO GET BETTER JUST AS MUCH AS YOU WANT TO HELP IT.

PART ONE
Birds

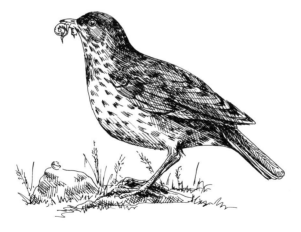

1

Rescue and Containment

Whether to rescue or to leave well alone

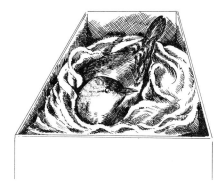

RESCUE SITUATIONS

The graphic, haunting pictures of birds struggling in the oil slicks that were created during the Gulf War told us all that the birds needed rescuing if they were to have any chance of survival. But it is not always that easy to assess a bird's situation and what may appear to be sickly or debilitated behaviour could be a natural part of a bird's daily routine.

I remember distinctly a wryneck that came into St Tiggywinkles displaying all the classic symptoms of torticollis – the spasms of the neck and head seen in many dying birds and typical of paramyxo virus infection in pigeons. This, however, is normal behaviour for a wryneck, hence its name, and it needed no help from me for any neck problem. But it *did* need rescuing, not because it showed any other signs of distress or injury but simply because it had been caught by a cat. Any bird that survives being caught by a predator, or is suspected of having escaped from a predator, should be treated with antibiotics (see Ch. 3, pp. 76–8) and observed for at least 48 hours before it is released.

Failure to get airborne

The wryneck, when rescued, was held captive by the cat so couldn't fly, but any free-living adult bird (with the possible exception of your friendly garden robin or the pigeons in Trafalgar Square) should fly off at any attempt to approach it – the flight response. If it makes no attempt to flee, fails to get airborne or only manages to fly for a short spell, then it probably needs to be rescued. But remember that this failure to get airborne will always be the case with swifts and any of the deep-diving aquatic birds such as grebes and divers, none of which can take off from land. They generally only need a helping hand, either into the air or onto a suitable stretch of water.

Swifts should be checked for injury and, if apparently sound, should be thrown as high as possible; this allows them to gather momentum and start circling to gather height. Always attempt this manoeuvre over grass just in case there is an unnoticed disability and the bird glides back to earth.

Divers and **grebes** need more specialised release techniques and should be handled with gloves, as they have sharp beaks which they will not hesitate to use. Your local birdwatching group or county bird recorder (listed in the *Birdwatcher's Yearbook*) will give advice on a suitable release site for each species.

Swans are renowned for landing in places where they are apparently unable to fly. They have invariably flown there but may have difficulty in flying out again – it's not that they are injured but simply that they need a considerable runway, both on water or land, in order to get airborne. They often land in fields to graze on a farmer's crop. If you are worried the swan may be trapped, be bold – try to touch one and watch it run then fly off. If it does not take off, however, it could well need rescuing, especially if there are power lines in the vicinity. Some swans end up landing on roads or walking into people's gardens or courtyards, where they keep all attempts at rescue by humans at bay. They do tend to be all 'puff and wind' and can be caught and released on a vacant stretch of water. I say 'vacant' because if that water is part of the territory of a pair of swans then your releasee could be in for trouble.

Many birds, not just swans, are found sitting on roads and will stay there, even if cars approach and pass them by. Once again, apart from the death-defying London pigeons who move for no one, any bird that does not fly off needs rescuing. If there is any doubt, turn around and have another look, just to make sure. Why not park the car safely and walk towards the bird, keeping yourself between it and the road so that if it attempts to flee it will not fall into the path of any passing traffic (which, incidentally, will hit you as well, if you are not very careful)? The bird may well fly off. Well and good, but if it cannot make a clean escape, it probably needs catching up and treating.

Road traffic causes many thousands of casualties every year. Far more numerous, though, are the juvenile birds that appear to need rescuing as they sit, lost and forlorn, around our gardens. Do not be fooled by their attitude, most of them are being cared for by their parents and will not need any help from us. They will eventually fly off with their parents and so should be left alone, except where they are in imminent danger or when they are obviously, and I mean obviously, injured. These so-called orphaned birds are a major problem every year, but as the majority are not injured and do not need help I do not propose to go into the rescue and rearing of orphans – a subject covered in my previous book, *The Complete Garden Bird*.

Crash landings and exhaustion
In September, when the baby bird season is drawing to its close, a new phenomenon occurs: crashes of **vagrant seabirds** into our gardens and onto our roads. These are not only gulls but also far more exotic species like auks, shearwaters, shags, petrels and even gannets. Often they will not, or in fact cannot, take off and need rescuing, but this entails nothing more than picking them up and taking them to the nearest stretch of coast for return to their natural marine habitat. Some will be exhausted and will need a few days to recover their strength, but don't keep any pelagic (ocean-going) bird for longer than necessary as they are susceptible to aspergillosis (see Ch. 2, p. 64), a fungal infection of their lungs and air-sacs.

It's mainly **seabirds**, **migratory birds** and **racing pigeons** that appear to suffer from exhaustion. The fate of many of the first mentioned was vividly illustrated to me on a return voyage from the USA when we witnessed all manner of birds trying to take refuge on the ship, even though we were thousands of miles from land. Some were unable to land and flew off towards who knows where; when we docked at

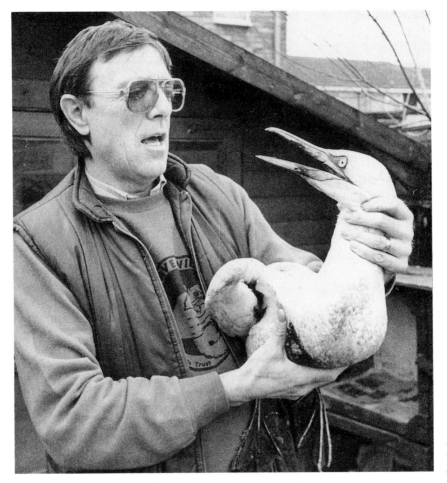

*A surprise visitor
– a crash-landed
gannet*

Southampton I found a tiny storm petrel that had obviously died trying to find shelter high on the forward poop deck.

Unlike these cases at sea, any bird over land that can manage to fly does not normally need help, but the bird with a drooping wing or a twisted, dangling leg *does* need our intervention (see Ch. 3). Birds with apparently only one leg probably have the other tucked up in their tummy feathers to keep it warm, but birds that cannot stand or which belly-flop to the ground have serious problems and are going to perish if you do not treat them; as is the bird that sits dejected and puffed out on your bird table making no attempt to feed. It probably has no strength left even to peck and this weakness is often the result of starvation and the downward spiral caused by prolonged severe cold or dry weather conditions.

Freezing weather and other hazards

Long spells of freezing weather have grave repercussions for fish-eating birds like **herons** and **kingfishers**, but watch out too for **ducks** or **swans** frozen to the ice. Try a few shouts and gesticulations and watch them waddle off. For your own safety always try long-range scaring tactics or a rope stretched from bank to bank before embarking on a very dangerous rescue over ice, which should never be attempted without getting help first.

Swans and **ducks** are large birds and always seem to be in trouble, especially where they clash with anglers. They are familiar to a lot of people, who soon notice the fishing line dangling from the beak, the float or spinner trailing behind or the ominous lump appearing in the swan's graceful neck. These birds have to be caught. Not too bad with a swan but almost impossible with a duck that can swim, dive, run or take off vertically to evade your desperate lunge with a net (see pp. 19–20).

ANY BIRD WITH LINE OR COTTON AROUND IT NEEDS ATTENTION AND SHOULD NOT BE RELEASED AGAIN UNTIL EVERY LAST VESTIGE OF THE LIGATURE HAS BEEN PAINSTAKINGLY REMOVED (see Ch. 4, pp. 91–2).

Oil on feathers

In addition to the situations outlined above, where rescues are necessary, there are those incidents which affect a bird's plumage, those crucial feathers that are a raincoat, an eiderdown and a means of flight. The merest drop of oil or paint opens the birds to a soaking and hypothermia, as has been so graphically illustrated by oil spill incidents. Any water bird with the slightest trace of oil on it needs specialised treatments (see Ch. 4, pp. 92–5) or else it will become waterlogged and succumb to hypothermia, whereas any land bird will drown if it falls into water.

Exotic escapes

One other situation that crops up quite regularly is the appearance of an exotic bird in the neighbourhood. These are nearly always escaped pets

Bird action

When to assist	*When to leave alone*
Bird cannot stand	Bird standing on one leg
One leg hangs useless	Apparently orphaned juvenile
Bird cannot fly	Bird can fly
Bird is a grounded swift	Apparently frozen in ice
Bird is a grounded grebe or diver	Swan grazing in field
Bird is an ocean-going species stranded inland	Any bird with only one eye except hawks
The beak is damaged	When you would endanger yourself or others
Bird has oil on its feathers	
Featherless orphan	
Bird standing on road	
Bird fallen in water	
Bird has fishing line or cotton on it	
Definitely frozen in ice	
Bird caught in trap (trapping is illegal)	
Bird is an exotic 'pet' species	
Bird of prey or swan confirmed as only having one leg or foot	

and can include parrots, lorikeets, budgerigars, canaries and even chickens. Make sure they are not glamorous, indigenous visitors like jays, hoopoes or waxwings, then try to entice them into the home until an owner can be found. Most of these birds would not survive wild in this country and could cause problems to native populations of more sensitive species by, for instance, commandeering likely nest sites.

Many birds are seen coping with apparently long-standing, serious disabilities and most can be left to survive naturally, even if they have only one eye or one leg or foot. Exceptions are swans or birds of prey, which cannot manage on only one leg; and whereas nearly all birds can manage with only one eye, the diurnal birds of prey would find it very difficult to catch their food. Catching birds of prey, however, is fraught with legal tripwires and you should contact the Department of the Environment, which may arrange for a suitable licence if necessary.

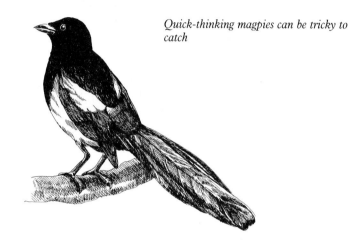

Quick-thinking magpies can be tricky to catch

THE CHASE AND CAPTURE

This is probably a misleading subheading, for the last thing you should do is chase a bird, and there is never any guarantee that you are going to capture it. However, birds are well known for their bird-brain intelligence and, apart from the quick-thinking magpies and other Corvids, should be easily outwitted and captured without a chase.

To chase a bird is not only taxing on your own fitness but can be harmful to the bird because it is stressful and can sometimes exacerbate any injuries. Most birds seem to register very little sensation of pain. Indeed, many of them, particularly black-headed gulls, will try to fly on broken wings, with the fractured bones piercing the skin and causing severe damage to surrounding soft tissue, muscle and ligaments. Chasing will only encourage them to do this, often making any treatment to save the wing difficult or even useless.

Try to treat your capture of a bird like an army manoeuvre, planning for all contingencies which, believe me, *will* rear their ugly heads.

Do not approach your bird immediately but stand, or preferably crouch, at a distance to assess its condition, wariness and ability to fly or run. Crouching and keeping low makes the bird less anxious than a hulking great body blotting out the skyline. Try not to look directly at the bird as this will simulate the action of a predator – a pair of staring eyes, to a bird, suggests a hawk, fox, owl or other hunter.

The bird will react instinctively to each of your movements and will seek an escape route. Close it off and offer an alternative escape route into a shed, building or blind alley. NEVER GIVE A CASUALTY THE CHANCE TO ESCAPE ONTO WATER OR A BUSY ROAD. Oiled birds on beaches are typical casualties where, unless they are approached from the direction of the sea, will head back onto the water, often to be lost for ever. And believe me it is much easier to catch a swan on land than it is on a lake or river.

Capturing with a net

Once you have your bird in sight, you have to capture it. Unless it is very debilitated it is very difficult simply to bend down and pick up a bird with the bare hand, especially if the bird is quite small and you are not used to handling such tiny, apparently frail creatures. If you need to pick up a small bird by hand, then hold it around the shoulders keeping the wings restrained close to the body. It may attempt to peck you but cannot cause any harm. It's far easier and more successful if you can use some form of net, or simply throw a *lightweight* coat or sweater over the bird. Fine for those who will occasionally be catching a sick bird; for those of you on 'call-outs' more regularly, it is worth investing in one of the various-sized **bird-catching nets** with padded rims that are available at many pet centres.

These will be suitable for smaller birds: sparrows, finches, robins and budgerigars, but for anything larger than a blackbird you should use a net that is at least 65cm across. In the absence of a purpose-made net, an angler's landing net with a long extending handle serves the purpose admirably. A pair of thick leather gloves will protect you from the bites and talons of larger birds or, as an alternative, the bird can be offered a towel to attack once you have it contained. Oil and paint may also contain residues that are harmful to you so a close-fitting pair of rubber or surgical gloves will offer protection.

Now concentrate on your bird, remembering that its instinctive reactions are much quicker than you can predict, so you must watch for even the slightest change of posture or flexing of a leg or wing. Watch the bird out of the corner of your eye and, keeping crouched, place your net in front of you about a half a metre off the ground. Then, very, very slowly start towards your bird, waiting after each step until the bird resettles. If it flexes its legs or defecates then it is definitely contemplating fleeing. Let it settle again. Try to move only as it looks away. Then, when you are sure you can net your bird instantly, bring the net down over the bird without hesitation and hold it down. Do not let go until you have approached the net and have the bird held securely through the fabric. Approaching and restraining quickly will prevent needless flapping and possibly more damage to the bird.

If the bird does manage to evade your lunge, do not chase it but wait until it settles and then start all over again.

The whole procedure of catching birds can be made much easier if there are two experienced handlers, the second of whom can distract the bird's attention and carry another net to cut off any escape attempt.

Capturing with a hook
Ducks and **swans** are in their element on water and as so many have had unhappy experiences of being beaten off by people with fishing rods and landing nets, they take one look at a net or a swan hook and glide into the distance. A **swan hook** is specially made for catching swans and has an attachment like a shepherd's crook at the end of a long pole. To a swan, however, it looks remarkably like a fishing rod. Hooked around the swan's neck it makes the bird's capture far less traumatic and I have been assured by a veterinary surgeon with a great deal of experience of swans that, if used properly, it can do no harm to the bird's very powerful neck.

Capturing by deception
Obviously, in heavily fished waters we cannot use either nets or hooks because many swans are wary of them, and we have to revert to the old ploy of deception: offer the swans small pieces of bread. Gradually

tempt them nearer and nearer then, when the injured bird is within arm's reach, make a lightning grab and grip it, by hand, just below the head. It will struggle, but pull it to you quickly, control its wings by tucking it under one arm or just pin it to the ground, keeping the wings under control at all times. Swans very seldom bite and even if they do they cannot hurt you. The last swan I had to catch had a damaged neck, so I even used its beak as a handhold as I pulled it ashore. (A swan's neck is so strong that even this manhandling did not cause any further damage to the injured neck.)

If you cannot manage the bread ploy, then a **swan on water** needs to be caught by a team in a boat. A rowing boat will not keep up with the swan, an outboard motor of at least 12hp is needed for a swift, short capture. Swans are fairly stable and not easily stressed, so a short sharp chase on water will not cause them any harm.

Ducks, on the other hand, are probably the most difficult of all birds to catch. They can swim, dive, run surprisingly fast and take off vertically from a standing start. When injured or in moult (eclipse) they usually cannot fly and can be approached.

The main type of call from members of the public alerting me to an injured duck are from those who have seen a bird wearing a glistening necklace of the plastic rings from the top of beer four-packs. They are often not a hindrance to the duck until they get snagged on an underwater branch or noosed onto a tree.

Bread is, once again, a very good ploy to tempt ducks onto land, where a lightning lunge with a net might just pre-empt a vertical take-off. On water, try deceiving the duck by keeping your net just below the surface and lifting as the duck swims over, tempted by the bread titbits.

In general it is against the law to take any wild bird, with the notable exception as allowed by Section IV, Paragraph (2)(a) of the Wildlife and Countryside Act 1981:

> A person shall not be guilty of an offence by reason of . . . the taking of any wild bird if he shows that the bird had been disabled otherwise than by his unlawful act and was taken solely for the purpose of tending it and releasing it when no longer disabled.

There are other sections dealing with illegal methods of taking wild birds but my view has always been that hand-held nets or hand-operated box traps for disabled birds are within the spirit of the law for those wishing to offer assistance to injured wild birds.

Hand-operated box traps

The use of a **hand-operated box trap** can be a lifesaver for an injured bird visiting your garden. Indeed, it is essential in the capture of disabled sparrows, pigeons and collared doves which, at the moment, do not enjoy the protection of the Wildlife and Countryside Act.

Quite simply, an inverted cardboard box is propped up at one end by a thin stick or garden cane about 30cm long. Attached to the bottom of the stick is a length of thin string, whose free end you take with you into the house or other suitable hiding place. Seed and other bird food is placed on the ground under the box then, as your injured bird ventures underneath, the stick is pulled away and the box, or even a basket, falls around the bird. To retrieve the bird, slide a tray underneath the box and take the whole lot inside the house. You can then reach in and take the bird out. If you remove the tray to look at the bird it will probably fly straight out and collide with a window in its efforts to escape.

Cardboard box trap

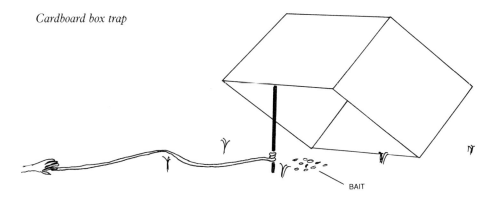

BAIT

Most cases of injured birds visiting your garden seem to be pigeons and collared doves. They can be legally caught in a special **pigeon cage trap**, which does them no harm and which is available from many game suppliers.

Birds trapped inside buildings

Birds uninjured but inside buildings do not normally need to be captured. Our method is to turn off all interior lighting and open all windows and doors, drawing the bird to the nearest exit. If this is not possible then wait until after dark, when the bird will roost and can be easily caught. Owls are different. They come alive in the dark and should be ambushed during the day rather than leaving doors and windows open all night. Birds I have had to release from buildings, other than the inevitable starling down the chimney, have included a little owl in a factory, a kestrel in a hospital, a pigeon in the county court, a pair of collared doves in a fast-fit exhaust centre and swifts in the voluminous roof of a stately home.

RESTRAINING AND CONTAINING YOUR BIRD

When your bird is eventually caught, you will need to handle it and contain it. Do not, at this stage, worry about its injuries, unless it cannot breathe, is bleeding profusely, is unconscious or soaking wet. These situations need prompt first aid (see Initial First Aid, pp. 31–5), but do not happen very often. All that is usually necessary on initial capture is to place the bird in a **warm**, **dark**, **secure cardboard box** and keep it **quiet** until you feel it has settled enough for you to assess its injuries. *Do not* give it anything to eat or drink at this stage.

Handling

The handling of all species of bird is very similar, with either one or both hands holding the shoulders of the bird to control its wings. Herons and swans will need to be tucked under one arm, with the legs of a heron held in one hand and its lethal beak in the other. A swan can be put into an open-ended sack with its neck and head out through a hole cut in the blind end.

Different birds have various characteristic methods of defending themselves and, although some efforts are futile, others, such as those employed by birds of prey and owls, can inflict serious injury. These birds attack feet first, only using their hooked beaks to bite as a last resort. It's always worth wearing gloves when handling small birds of prey but even gloves will not protect you against the larger species: eagles, goshawks, large owls and falcons, which should only be handled

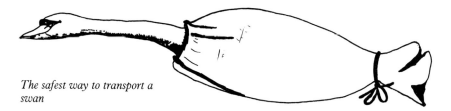

The safest way to transport a swan

by experts who will know how to control the bird's legs and avoid contact with those dangerous talons. If in any doubt, throw a blanket or jacket around the bird and wrap it up, taking special care that the feet are not exposed, even for an instant.

Crows, cormorants and gulls will bite and herons, bitterns, divers and gannets may well attempt to spear your eyes. In the case of the former species, wrap a strong elastic band around the beak, making sure the bird can still breathe through the nares (nostrils) at the top of its beak. (Incidentally, gannets do not have external nostrils so their beaks should never be held closed for any length of time.)

The sharp-beaked fishing birds should have their heads controlled at all times or, even better, covered with a towel. But always be prepared for that lightning-quick jab.

All birds, even the tiny ones, will attempt to bite or defend themselves. Many cannot hurt you but sometimes the surprise of a sudden nip may make you drop your casualty, and you will have to start the chase and capture all over again.

ONE WORD OF WARNING: NEVER LET ANY BIRD, NO MATTER WHAT SIZE, ANYWHERE NEAR YOUR FACE. I have had a sparrow bite my nose in an unguarded moment and an owl grab my ear as it passed by. It hurts, and can cause serious injury if an eye is involved.

When handling any animal, birds included, concentrate at all times. Give them the benefit of the doubt. Their reaction time is far quicker than yours and they will strike, given half a chance.

The ABC of first aid

A Airways – make sure the airways are clear
B Breathing – make sure the casualty is breathing
C Circulation – make sure the heart is beating and blood circulating

---

TRANSPORTING YOUR CASUALTY

Most casualties are caught or rescued away from your house or care facility. It's not good enough simply to release them into a hedge or onto a stream. If you have managed to catch a bird, that bird needs care and attention, first aid and possibly more intensive treatment. Make sure it's stable and get it to more intensive care as quickly as possible.

Boxes

Cardboard boxes with lids are ideal for carrying most birds, except perhaps for the very small or the very large. An old towel on the bottom will give the bird a steadier footing and a few air holes punched around the bottom will give ventilation without the bird being able to see out. A cold or wet bird could be wrapped in a 'space blanket' or one similar to those given to marathon runners when they have finished a course. This will help to retain crucial body heat, which is essential because every bird casualty will go into some form of shock.

Bags

Small birds can be carried in small cloth bags, whereas long birds, like pheasants, are quite comfortable in a zip-up holdall, even with their tail feathers poking out of one end.

The prime consideration in transporting is to keep the bird subdued by confining it in the dark and to resist the temptation to peek into the container until you have reached your destination.

It's not wise to carry any bird loose in a car. If it is aware, it will try to get out through a window and could be a great hazard both to itself and the driver, especially if it disappears behind any panelling.

RECORD KEEPING

A lot of information and experience about wildlife casualties has been lost simply because the details were not written down as they occurred. At St Tiggywinkles many patients come in displaying diverse problems, and it is very helpful to be able to look back at the records of previous patients with similar problems, to see whether we had success or failure from a particular treatment. We also publish that information in various forms so that others can learn from our experiences. It is sad to know that some once very active wildlife rehabilitators have either died or retired without leaving the benefit of their knowledge behind, no matter how insignificant it may have seemed to them. Even the ups and downs of just one casualty could help another if its history had been published. We publish a newsletter called *Hands On*, in which we aim to spread the word about rehabilitation. In it we invite contributions, no matter how small, from all rescuers. A few lines of experience could save the life of an animal.

But, back to record keeping. As you can see, I believe that a record card is essential, like the one illustrated opposite. On it should be recorded the date, name of the species and sex if known. The finder's name and address gives a valuable record of the source of that animal, especially if it is a protected species. Some birds, listed in the Wildlife and Countryside Act under Schedule IV, should be handed to a Licensed Rehabilitation Keeper who will fill in the requisite Department of the Environment records. As you become more *au fait* with wildlife casualties you will come across more and more legislation. In order to simplify things for you, I have listed the regulations that apply to wildlife later in this book (see Appendix III, p. 203). It would be a good idea to become familiar with the laws which, in the main, actually favour the helping of the sick or injured wild animal or bird.

Your record card could also give some details of where the casualty was found and the circumstances of its rescue – some need to be released back in home territory.

Other information could include the weight of the casualty, which is a good yardstick for measuring its progress while it is with you, as well as being a possible diagnostic aid if the bird is grossly underweight for its species. References to the normal weight for most British birds can be found in *The Handbook of Birds of Europe, the Middle East and North Africa*. A quick check can be made by feeling the bird's breast bone, which should be well padded with muscle. If it feels sharp and prominent, the bird has lost weight for some reason. Symptoms, of course, are important, as are details of any treatments or food and drink it has been given. Never give brandy or milk, which have damaging effects: brandy will depress a bird's metabolism, and they find the lactose in milk totally indigestible.

A regime of treatment and then records of application of medica-
ments are essential. The medical record will be especially helpful to
your vet in monitoring your casualty's progress. And a record of any
ectoparasites (external parasites) may well assist future enquiries from
zoologists and the like.

Finally, there is the outcome: either release or death; and do not be
too distressed if it is the latter. It happens. I always say that any wild bird
or animal that allows itself to be caught is probably dying. If we can help
it live then we have done our best. If it dies we have still done our best
but perhaps we have learnt something that will help the next casualty
with similar problems – the filed record card will give you that
information.

ST TIGGYWINKLES RECORD CARD

Date			No.	

Name of Finder	Circumstances of Rescue
Address	

Preliminary Diagnosis	Daily Record Diet

Weight	Approx Age
Sex	Bead Marking
External Parasites	

Daily Record / Diet table:

Date	Wt	Med	Fed	Date	Wt	Med	Fed

Tests

Faeces	Skin	Blood PCV	Wounds	Fungus

Confirmed Diagnosis
Treatment

Outcome

27

INITIAL HOUSING

The most frequent cause of panic, both for a rescued bird and its finder, is when the casualty is apparently in the security of a home and is being transferred from a carrying box to more suitable housing. When the bird sees light, as the lid is opened, it makes a frantic dash for freedom and often escapes, only to fall foul of the hazards to be found in a house: a window, a bowl of washing-up water, a small gap under the kitchen cupboard, or even a cat. All are potential dangers and should be taken into account before opening the box. As an added precaution against losing the bird completely, just check that all windows and doors are closed and that windows are covered if possible, or else, in its headlong flight for freedom, your bird could collide with the glass and add concussion to its other problems.

My preferred way of removing any bird from a box is to put on a glove and slide my hand into a gap in the lid, keeping it tight around my arm. Then I feel for the bird and only when I have it securely do I open the lid and remove the bird for transfer to a more suitable container.

Cardboard boxes
If there is nothing more suitable, the casualty can be kept in a cardboard box lined on the bottom with newspaper covered once again with an old towel to give the bird's feet some purchase. For a perching bird a log or branch can be laid on the bottom to make sitting more comfortable. Overall, the container should be kept warm, at least 30°C, and *almost* dark. If it is completely blacked out, the bird will simply sleep, whereas to improve its chances of recovery we want it to drink and feed as early as possible.

Cages
Bird cages are not suitable containers for wild birds, except for those breeding cages where all but one side is solid wood. Even then, the wired side should be partially covered with a towel to deter the bird from battering itself against the bars in its efforts to escape.

NEVER EVER USE HAY OR STRAW IN BIRD CAGES. Hay and straw tend to be host to fungus spores than can be fatal to all birds. Newspaper or paper towels and a perch or two are all that is necessary.

PROVIDING FOOD AND DRINK

I mention that the bird should drink and feed as soon as possible. That's very true, but water, especially in drinking containers, is a real hazard to an injured bird. Only ever put drinking containers – and they must be low-sided – in with a bird if it can stand and has complete control. Even then, a budgie's gravity-fed 'water fountain' is far safer than a bowl as the bird cannot possibly fall into it. The bird may, however, need to be shown how to use it by your dunking its beak.

If you have no other equipment, you can dunk the bird's beak in a bowl of Lectade or rehydrating fluid (see below). A Lectade (Beechams) solution should also be put into the water fountain (it is preferable to plain water, especially for a dehydrated bird). If that is not available the home-made International Rehydrating Fluid is perfectly suitable. This can be mixed up, as required, to the following formula, which should be replaced after 24 hours:

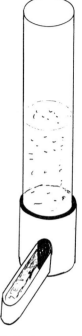

Budgerigar water fountain

International Rehydrating Fluid (isotonic)

1 tablespoon of sugar
1 teaspoon of salt
1 litre warm water

Food suitable for the species – insectivorous, seed- or fish-eating – should also be made available. It is always a good barometer of a bird's condition – if it starts feeding, then it has taken the first step to recovery. But *be careful* with any of the live foods such as maggots or mealworms, as they may well attack a seriously debilitated bird.

PROVIDING WARMTH

Warmth is the prime agent in healing sick or injured birds. It can be provided with a hot water bottle covered with an old towel or by placing the bird's container on a radiator or in an airing cupboard. Both methods are all right as a temporary measure, but be careful not to let the bird overheat (see Hyperthermia, Ch. 2, pp. 59–60). Far more reliable are the various electric devices available.

There are **ceramic heat lamps** that emit no light, only heat. One of these can be suspended over a sick bird, but owing to their size – 100 watts and 150 watts – they are only really suitable over open pens for larger birds that cannot fly. Ducks and birds of that size can be kept in a lobster-pot type playpen with wire mesh over the top to prevent them flying. Either a ceramic lamp or an electric heat mat will provide enough warmth. Swans are too large even for a playpen but can be kept in a shed or utility room on plenty of newspapers – the order of the day for all the larger birds.

For smaller birds, one of the commercially made, thermostatically controlled **hospital cages** will provide ideal recuperative accommodation for birds sized from a wren to a pigeon.

Birds that have difficulty supporting themselves can be placed on an old towel rolled into a horseshoe shape. Then, when they are settled, their bowls of food and shallow water or rehydrating fluid can be put within reach.

ANY BIRD, NO MATTER WHAT ITS OBVIOUS INJURY, COULD BE THE CARRIER OF INFECTION TO OTHER BIRDS SO ISOLATE ANY NEWCOMERS FOR AT LEAST 24 HOURS. I find, however, that small birds up to collared dove size fare much better if put with birds of a similar size and disposition and although the isolation of disease is the recommended procedure, I have had no known incident of one disease passed to another bird.

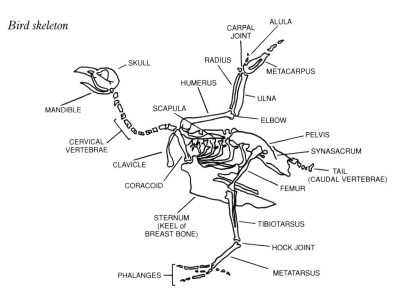

Bird skeleton

Obviously, predatory birds should not be placed with subordinate species and aggressive species like male blackbirds and robins should be kept separate from their own kind or else the outcome may be the humdinger of a battle.

INITIAL FIRST AID

With any new bird casualty it's always advisable to leave it warm and comfortable for 24 hours or the stress of being handled can kill it. There are, however, some conditions and situations that demand immediate attention. Most important of all, check whether anything is life threatening:

1 Can the bird breathe?
Make sure its neck is extended and then clean away anything blocking its mouth, nostrils (nares) and on the inside of its mouth, using a cotton bud.

2 Is the bird bleeding?
If it is, place a pad of clean gauze on the haemorrhage site and apply pressure for a minute or two. Slight bleeding can often be halted with a haemostat-like caustic pencil or diluted potassium permanganate, available from chemists. Bleeding vessels or feather stubs can be controlled using artery forceps and, if necessary, can be ligatured with catgut (see Ch. 3, pp. 71–5).

3 Is the bird unconscious?
If in doubt as to whether the bird is dead or merely unconscious, give it the benefit of the doubt and treat it accordingly. An unconscious bird should be supported upright, on its keel (breast bone). It should be kept warm and *not* be offered anything to drink. A vet can prescribe an injection of corticosteroids, dexamethasone, to alleviate both inflammation and stress.

4 Is the bird soaking wet?
Hold it upside down for a few seconds in case there is any fluid in its trachea. Then dry it as much as possible with a warm towel and place in a box in a warm place or in a special heat box or cage without delay.

5 *Are its eyes damaged or not able to close?*

Damaged eyes should be treated immediately with bland chloramphenicol eye ointment, available from a vet, applied along the lower lids. An early assessment of the damage by a vet experienced in bird ophthalmology may save the bird's vital sight.

Eyes that are permanently open because the bird is unconscious should be moistened either several times daily with hypromellose drops or once daily with the longer-lasting Lacri-Lube ointment, available from most chemists.

6 *Are there fractures of the wings, legs or beak?*

Any fractures should be initially stabilised for at least 24 hours, when a more detailed assessment and treatment can be instigated.

Broken wings These can be lightly strapped to the bird's body using non-adhesive cohesive bandage, which is available from Boots and other chemists. This arrangement will prevent any further damage until the injury can be assessed and splinted accordingly. Fold the wing alongside the body in as natural a position as possible. Pass the bandage over the injured wing and under the body in front of the leg, across and then up and over the other side of the body behind the other leg. The bandage is then passed under the back of the good wing, over the back and down over the rear of the injured wing, behind that leg and across and up in front of the other leg, avoiding the leading edge of the good wing. The end is then passed over the back to join in a figure of eight.

Points to look out for are that the bandage is not too tight and that it crosses underneath over the breast bone (which can be felt between and slightly forward of the legs). The uninjured wing and both legs should be free of all restraints.

This method of bandaging allows the bird to stand and balance although it may take a few hours to get used to the restriction on the broken wing.

Any wounds on the wing should be bathed with dilute Savlon (or preferably Hibiscrub) (see Ch. 2, p. 47) and covered with a non-adhesive dressing before any strapping is applied. Non-adhesive dressings, such as Melolin, are available from Boots and other chemists.

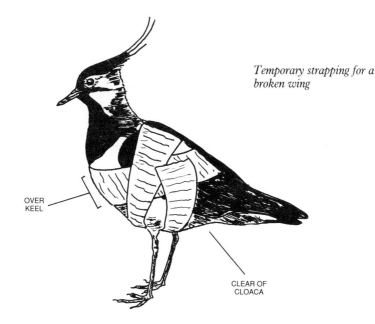

Temporary strapping for a broken wing

OVER KEEL

CLEAR OF CLOACA

Elastic or crepe bandage should *never* be used for strapping as they may cause constriction. Also out of bounds on bird wings are adhesive tapes, which will inevitably damage feathers as they are removed. (See also Ch. 3, pp. 83–5.)

Broken legs A leg that is simply hanging rather than being dragged is more than likely fractured. Often by feeling along the point where the bird loses control of its leg, you will be able to locate the crepitus, where the two bone fragments are touching. Birds appear to have little sensation of pain and will, in many instances, think nothing of trying to walk on a broken leg or flap a broken wing, causing all manner of damage to the surrounding tissues. Hence the need for stabilisation of the fracture before the bird can do more damage to itself. If you are careful while you are handling a fracture site you will cause hardly any discomfort to the bird and can set about lining up the injured limb and strapping it in place.

I like to deal with fractured legs as soon as they arrive because I know full well that as soon as I turn my back my casualty will try to walk.

Lay the bird on its side with the injured leg uppermost. Cover its head with a towel and, if possible, get somebody else to hold the bird quietly. Now line the fracture site up by pulling slightly to make sure the two bone ends don't overlap (reducing the fracture). Take the time to make sure the toes are pointing in the same direction as the opposite foot – it's all too easy to get it wrong at this stage.

Alongside the fracture site apply a splint that is the same length as that part of the bird's leg. Strips of wood sliced from bamboo or ice-cream sticks are ideal and can be trimmed to any size. Now wrap the leg and splint with strips of zinc oxide plaster, making sure not to pull it too tight and impede the leg's circulation. Finally, flex the leg to 90° at the hock (tibiotarsal) joint and hold it at right angles with a diagonal strip of zinc oxide plaster. Now, in indelible pen, write on the strapping the date the splint was applied. This will remind you to remove the splint in 7 to 10 days when the fracture should have set. If it hasn't set by then re-splint the fracture for another 5 days, but do not bother to flex the hock joint again.

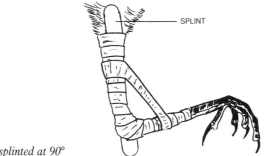

Broken leg splinted at 90°

Pigeons, for some unknown reason, are always breaking their legs. The pigeon-racing fraternity has even designed a clip-on plastic splint which is ideal for many other bird species. Called the 'Columbo-clip' it can simply be clamped around the reduced fracture and held in place with two clips, and taken off in 7 days and refitted if necessary (see also Ch. 2, pp. 79–82).

Beak fractures Broken beaks will deteriorate if not stabilised immediately. The simplest temporary method is just to hold the beak in a closed position and wrap it with zinc oxide plaster, making sure to avoid the nostrils (nares). In fact, if the bird has any trouble breathing then strap the beak slightly open using a piece of wood as a wedge. As I said before, gannets have no nares, and so should always have their beaks wedged open.

7 Is the bird caught up in fishing line, cotton etc?

Any form of ligature formed by any type of line should be removed *immediately* and *completely*. I find it an advantage to work under a magnifying lamp because I often have to search any wounds very carefully for telltale remnants of line. If you do not cut it, then it's sometimes possible to unravel it all in one piece. There is often a lot of bleeding when the line is removed from a bird's feet or legs. Once the wounds have been cleaned, the haemorrhage can usually be stopped with pressure pads of clean gauze.

If the bird has fishing line coming out of its mouth then *do not cut it*. Instead, clamp the end of the line securely with forceps or tie it to a pair of scissors. This will make it much easier to remove it in its entirety (see Ch. 4, pp. 91–2).

8 Other conditions requiring immediate first aid

The only other common conditions that call for urgent attention are that of an oiled bird (see Ch. 4, pp. 92–5) and those caught by cats. Prior to the more involved fluid therapy (see below), the eyes, beaks and mouths of an oiled bird should be cleaned with a cloth or swabbed, and a catted bird should have an injection of antibiotics (see Ch. 3, pp. 76–8).

IT'S ALWAYS BETTER TO LEAVE ANY CASUALTY FOR A SETTLING-IN PERIOD BUT NEVER TAKE THIS AS MATTER OF FACT AND ASSESS EACH AND EVERY CASUALTY TO DECIDE WHETHER IT DOES NEED EARLIER ATTENTION.

FLUID THERAPY

Slightly more advanced in terms of technique than the other aspects of initial first aid, but possibly the most crucial life-saver, is the replacement of the inevitable loss of body fluids. About 70% of an animal's body weight is water in various forms, both inside the body cells (intracellular) and outside (extracellular). Extracellular fluid includes the blood and other obvious body liquids, like the aqueous humour of the eye and the moisture on the mucous membranes in the mouth. Normally, body water is being lost all the time, especially through respiration and excretion. Equally normally, this loss is replaced by drinking and feeding. If it is not replaced then dehydration gradually increases, resulting in the death of cells and the life-threatening condition of hypovolemic shock, which occurs when the loss of body fluids can be as little as 12–15%.

An injured or sick wild bird may not have been able to drink and feed and will not have replaced the natural wastage of fluids from both the intracellular and extracellular reservoirs. However, a bird that is bleeding or has diarrhoea will lose its fluids more rapidly, straight from the reservoir of extracellular fluids which are made up of water, electrolytes, sodium and potassium. The last two chemicals are vital to the cell function of the body and they control the removal of waste products. Without the latter function, waste soon accumulates in the body, causing toxic reactions and, ultimately, cell deaths.

The primary aim of fluid therapy in countering dehydration is to replace the fluids that have been lost with a similar compound to a similar volume. Blood lost cannot be replaced in birds, but if the deficit is made up with fluids, the natural function of blood replacement may cope with the problem.

There are many complex types of fluid available for replacement, but many veterinary practices carry the two most suitable for use in birds. The first, commonly known as dextrose/saline, contains 4% dextrose and 0.18% sodium chloride and is useful to replace primary water loss from both reservoirs. The rapid loss of water and electrolytes through bleeding or diarrhoea can be replaced by Hartmann's Solution.

Under a veterinary surgeon's instruction, these replacements can be given either intravenously, the preferred route, or subcutaneously, which unfortunately will have little immediate effect on the shocked patient.

ALL FLUIDS SHOULD BE WARMED TO BODY TEMPERATURE – IN A BIRD THIS IS ABOUT 40°C – BEFORE BEING GIVEN.

More effective than the subcutaneous route is the administration of fluids by the mouth, with the preferred proprietary mix being Lectade (Beechams), available from veterinary centres. In the event of this not being available, then the home-made International Rehydrating Fluid (see Ch. 1, p. 29) will suffice until Lectade can be obtained. MOST

OTHER FLUIDS, I.E. WATER, BRANDY, MILK, SCOTCH OR GIN, WILL HARM
THE DEHYDRATED BIRD AND SHOULD NOT BE GIVEN.

HOW MUCH FLUID SHOULD BE GIVEN?

You should aim to replace like with like and volume with the same
volume. The losses incurred by bleeding or diarrhoea can be estimated
from the amounts seen to be lost. General dehydration, which is the
commonest emergency found in birds, can be calculated on the estimated degree of dehydration multiplied by the bird's body weight, plus
a daily maintenance amount equivalent to the bird's normal daily loss of
fluids through expiration and excretion. A bird could be given maintenance fluids at the rate of 50 millilitres per kilogram of body weight
every 24 hours.

The degree of dehydration can be roughly estimated by clinical signs
which, in a bird, would be the following:

Estimate of dehydration in birds	
Clinical signs	*Estimated degree of dehydration*
No obvious changes but assume all injured birds have some fluid deficit.	up to 5%
Skin appears tight, especially over the keel (breast bone).	5–6%
The skin forms temporary tents if pulled up. The eyes look dull. The inside of the mouth is dry, not moist as is usual.	7–10%
The mouth is very dry. The feet and wing tips are cold. The skin stays tented if it's pulled up. The heartbeat is rapid and the bird looks ill, listless and depressed.	10–12%
The bird is near death. Not moving. It feels cold as shock sets in.	12–15%

A simple calculation on a 300g pigeon that had flown into a window and which had an estimated percentage of dehydration of 10% would be:

Fluid deficit 300g $\times$ 0.10 = 30ml

Maintenance at 50ml/kg per day = 15ml

Therefore the pigeon needs 15ml of fluid every day, together with 30ml of fluid over the first two days to replace the deficit.

HOW TO GIVE FLUIDS

Giving fluids to pigeons is probably the most rewarding act of first aid *and* the easiest. All the pigeon family, the Columbiformes, have, unlike other British birds, the ability to suck fluids up through their beaks. Offering an injured pigeon or dove a cup of Lectade held to its beak usually results in it being most gratefully taken in with great gulps. Giving fluids to any other species may involve the slight complication of administration by crop or stomach tube.

I know this suggestion reeks of force-feeding suffragettes, or geese for pâté de fois gras, but if it is done properly and carefully, with a little practice, 'gavage', as it is known, can save many lives.

In short, a round-ended tube is passed down the bird's throat into its stomach, the proventriculus, at the bottom of the oesophagus (gullet).

Different sized birds need various sizes of tubes, ranging from a 4-inch stainless steel Spreull's needle for small birds to a Lan-am feeder, a large form of syringe, for pigeons and owls, and various thicknesses and lengths of soft rubber tubing for larger species. Attached to the tubes are various sizes of syringe, which are used to measure the amount of fluids given. A tiny bird may only need a 1ml or 2ml syringe, whereas a swan could require a 60ml syringe filled three times. Unfortunately, there are no recommended amounts for individual species, so each administration should be closely monitored in case fluid backs up the throat to the glottis and the bird's respiratory system. If that does happen, keep the bird's head high and see if it can swallow and sort out the crisis for itself. Alternatively, hold the bird upside down for a few seconds to let any fluid drain from the trachea (wind pipe).

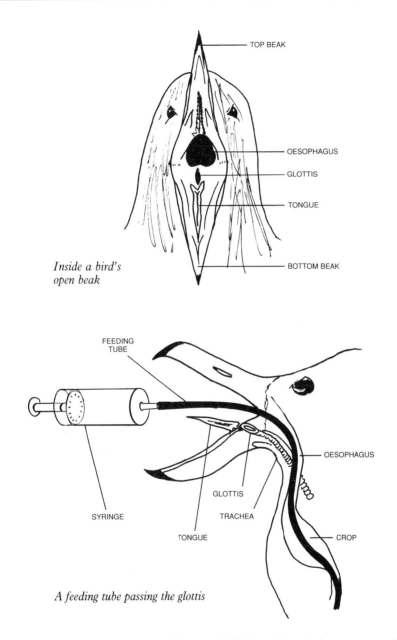

Inside a bird's open beak

TOP BEAK

OESOPHAGUS

GLOTTIS

TONGUE

BOTTOM BEAK

FEEDING TUBE

SYRINGE

TONGUE

GLOTTIS

TRACHEA

OESOPHAGUS

CROP

A feeding tube passing the glottis

I would recommend that tubing a bird should only be attempted if there are two people available: one who holds the bird with its neck extended and beak wide open, and the other who slides in the tube and

39

gives the fluids. An overhead light will help you to locate the glottis and any overflow of liquids.

To calculate the length of tube likely to be needed to reach the proventriculus, hold the tube from the end of the beak along the contours of the neck and body to a point just below the breast bone, where the proventriculus ends and the gizzard begins. Coat the rounded end of the tube with a little lubricant like KY jelly or liquid paraffin and slide it down the throat to the side of the glottis.

As the tube slides down the throat into the crop it may well encounter some resistance. Do not push, but gently rotate the tube and allow it to proceed under its own weight. When you are satisfied that the next resistance you feel is the gizzard, at the end of the proventriculus, gradually enter the measured amount of fluid from the syringe attached to the free end of the tube, all the time watching for that dangerous overflow of liquid into the throat and glottis.

When all the fluid has been given, do not remove the syringe from the tube, but pull both it and the tube out of the throat. The bird's head may need to be supported above its body to prevent any liquid running back into the throat.

I would recommend that any newcomer to the procedure receive practical instruction of how to gavage from an experienced person, but as this is not standard veterinary practice it may be necessary to get advice from the nearest wildlife rescue centre.

After fluid therapy of any sort, the bird should show an improvement and may be inclined to take its own fluids. By all means let it do this, but make sure that the original deficit, planned to be replaced over two days, has been given. Maintenance fluids can be stopped once the bird is drinking normally.

2

Assessment and Treatment of Injuries

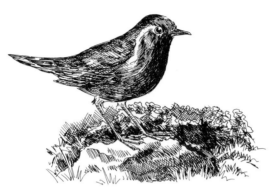

In spite of even the most sophisticated first-aid measures some birds are going to die during the first 24 hours of confinement. A bird's metabolism is highly tuned, working at a much faster rate than those of most mammals. They react much faster than mammals, heal much more efficiently and quickly and also, I'm afraid, turn off and die just as quickly. I always think that a bird has the ability to choose to switch off its life support and just expire. I have seen it happen in an instant, especially amongst injured pheasants and ospreys, which will sometimes simply die in your hands before you have time even to think of first aid. Although we are all trying to make those first 24 hours more reliable, I feel that we do have to be prepared for those early fatalities, but we must not let them deter us in our efforts to save others.

Those that do survive the initial admittance into care and settle in their cardboard boxes or hospital cages should, after 24 hours, be thoroughly examined for injury or disease. But just remember that there may be more than one thing wrong with the casualty, so check over the whole bird each time, even though a broken leg, wing or beak or some other obvious injury may be staring you in the face.

INITIAL ASSESSMENT

A bird's overall attitude and appearance can give many clues to its condition and general disposition. So before you pick up the bird for examination, take a peek at it and note the bird's attitude toward you. Notice whether it is standing up; is it only using one leg because the other is injured or is it merely resting? Do its eyes appear bright; is it aware of its surroundings or does it appear depressed, listless and uninterested? Most important of all, does it show fear or aggression at your approach? A bird that shows no response is probably still suffering from dehydration (see Ch. 1, pp. 35–7) or shock, whereas a bird that pecks you is feeling much better.

Keep a check list of all the points you notice or, alternatively, have a pre-printed schedule of points to look for with each casualty. Every out-of-the-ordinary feature you record gives a clue to the problems the bird is experiencing, although each clue could lead to various diagnoses. For instance, a bird that is not standing could be weak, low in vitamins, concussed, poisoned or simply just have two broken legs. So each clue may not provide the answer immediately but could well be a guide to the next stage of the assessment.

Some information, like the circumstances of the rescue, will give you a vital lead into the condition of the bird and should be asked of the rescuer and included on your check list. The first stage of your check list can be completed even before the bird is examined and could include the headings in the boxes on the next two pages.

EXAMINATION OF THE BIRD IN THE HAND

Armed with the answers to the previous two sets of questions, you will have some leads when it comes to examining the bird more closely. Once again, work to a check list and leave no feather unturned as you check every inch of the bird.

Weight
If at all possible it would help to weigh the bird, to assess its progress and to calculate dose rates for medicines. Take the weight in grams using electronic kitchen scales. The feathering does tend to make a bird

Questions for the rescuer

Was the bird found on or near a road?	If yes, look for concussion, fractures and eye damage.
Was the bird caught by a cat?	Even suspicion is enough to suggest septicaemia, needing treatment with antibiotics (see Ch. 3, pp. 76–8). Look for skin tears, eye damage or balloon-like swellings of the skin (subcutaneous emphysema, see p. 66).
Was the bird caught in cotton or line?	Check any deep wounds for more line. Wounds may need suturing (see Ch. 3, pp. 72–4). Check for dehydration.
Was the bird found under a window or patio door?	Will probably have concussion and some cranial haemorrhage.
Was the bird found under power lines?	Look for fractures, skin tears, abrasions and, in particular, damage to wings, beak and head.
Is there a suspicion of gunshot wounds?	Check all over for matted feathers covering a wound. Get it X-rayed. (See Ch. 3, pp. 78–9.)
Is there any history of crop spraying or insecticide used in the area?	Flaccid paralysis or, the opposite, chronic seizures, could well be the result of chemical poisoning (see Ch. 4, pp. 96–8).

look larger than it is, making estimates of its weight impractical (see Ch. 3, pp. 77–8).

Wings
Extend both wings, looking and feeling for fractures, dislocations, skin tears, subcutaneous emphysema (swelling) around the shoulders, and any damage to the main feathers. Each wing, if healthy, should automatically spring back into place alongside the body.

Assessment of the bird itself

Is the bird able to stand without assistance?	If not, look for concussion, vitamin deficiency (possible in ducks and swans fed on a bread diet), two broken legs, poisoning (particularly in gulls and waterfowl), and suspect general weakness and dehydration.
Is the bird only standing on one of its legs?	Take a note of which leg and check the other for fractures, ligatures, dislocations, frost damage and subcutaneous emphysema (swelling) around the hip. There may be a sprain.
Are either of the wings drooping?	Check the injured wing for fractures, dislocations, skin tears, ligatures, subcutaneous emphysema around the shoulder, or just a sprain.
Is the head being held straight and upright?	If not, look for concussion, or subcutaneous emphysema around the back of the neck. There could be an inner ear infection (see pp. 50–1). Or is it a species with peculiar head movements like the wryneck or barn owl?
Are both its eyes closed?	Look for concussion, eye infection, dehydration, mites, sinusitis (moisture from the nostrils), or general weakness.
Is just one eye closed?	Possibly infection, sinusitis or concussion, but be aware of one-eyed colds and ornithosis (see Ch. 4, p. 98) in Columbiformes (doves, pigeons etc.). It may be worth having a vet test for ornithosis if there is any doubt.

Continued on page 45.

| Does the bird breathe with its beak open? | Possibly stress or overheating. Look for trichomoniasis (see pp. 66–8), syngamus worms (see p. 51), beak damage or a respiratory infection, especially aspergillosis in sea birds. |
| Do its feathers seem puffed up? | Could be hypothermia or illness. Feather mites are another possibility. Something is wrong. |

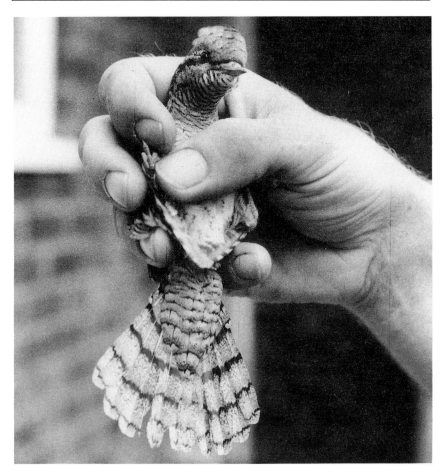

Examine every casualty thoroughly – there may be more than one injury

Legs

Look and feel along each leg for fractures, dislocations, ligatures and swellings on the joints or feet. Check for broken toes and swelling underneath the feet.

Beak

The beak should be solid – check for fractures. It should line up at the sides (except in crossbills) and not be over length. If in doubt, refer to an illustrated book on birds.

Mouth

Open the beak and check that the mucous membranes are moist and pink. If dry or pale, treat for dehydration (see Ch. 1, pp. 35–40). Look at the back of the throat for trichomoniasis (see pp. 66–8) and in the glottis and trachea for syngamus worms (see p. 64). The back of the throat may contain other worm types (see Endoparasites, p. 51). Check the tongue is clear and undamaged, especially the over-long tongues of woodpeckers. Water birds may have leeches in the slots in the roof of the mouth (choanae) through which air passes to the glottis. Birds do not have teeth, but many species have serrated, sharp edges to their beaks.

Nares (nostrils)

Wipe the nostrils with a cotton bud. Remove any leeches found in water birds with a pair of tweezers.

Eyes

Both eyes should be the same diameter, with the lids and nictitating membrane, the third eyelids (see p. 52), keeping them moist. Look for damage to the front of the eye, swellings around the eye which could be damage or infection. Mites may also cause eye problems. Water birds may have leeches tucked under the eyelids. Rapid vibration of the eyes may be a condition known as nystagmus, caused by concussive injuries.

Ears

These are simple sockets under the feathers behind the eyes and are at different levels in owls. Check for infectious discharge, ear mites or bleeding. (See also pp. 50–1.)

Crop

Feel the crop (throat) for food content and if a hard, unmoving nodule is present suspect trichomoniasis. Sometimes bread or large pieces of food like acorns will cause a blockage, but these will be palpable.

Keel, sternum or breast bone

The sternum should be well padded on both sides by a muscle mass. If it feels sharp and thin, then suspect starvation. Possible causes are beak damage, fishing line, trichomoniasis infection, a blocked alimentary canal, or either very cold or very dry weather, when food is hard to find.

Cloaca

Birds have only one orifice of excretion and reproduction, just below the base of the tail. Check it is clean and tight. If it is soiled the bird may not have been able to stand for some time, which may lead to cloacitis (see pp. 48–9). Hard swellings may be egg-binding (see p. 51).

Feathers

Look for broken feathers or matting of the close body feathers, usually suggesting a hidden wound. (See also shot wounds, Ch. 3, pp. 78–9; feather lice, p. 55; and oiled birds, Ch. 4, pp. 92–5.)

SPECIFIC CONDITIONS (in alphabetical order)

After you have checked the bird thoroughly, some conditions and injuries will have come to light. Other than the more involved conditions discussed in chapters 3 and 4, the following are problems commonly encountered in wild bird casualties.

Abrasions

Most wounds where the skin has not been seriously interrupted should be cleaned with dilute Savlon or Hibiscrub. Use pads of cotton wool and leave the wounds uncovered. No further treatment should be necessary.

Disinfectant solution for bathing wounds

Add enough Savlon or Hibiscrub, to clear warm water, to colour it. A
   strong solution is not necessary.

Abscesses (see Ch. 3, p. 78)

Aspergillosis (see Respiratory infection, below)

Beak damage

There are normally two types of damage to beaks – either part or all of the beak is missing, or else it is fractured. Broken beaks are dealt with in chapter 3. Missing beaks or parts of beaks can be dealt with in various, but always innovative, ways. I have seen many birds cope without a top beak but those missing a lower beak face great difficulties, especially with their tongues.

There have been heroic attempts at prostheses for both top and lower beaks, some successful and some dismal failures. A local dentist may be persuaded to have a go; it's sometimes the only chance a bird has and the prosthesis has to be tailored to suit each individual. If you want a template of a beak shape, then the British Museum, (Natural History) Ornithology Section at Tring, Hertfordshire, and possibly your local museum, will have 'skins' and skeletons of all British species.

Some waders, particularly woodcocks, have sensitive tips to their beaks which are essential to their lifestyle, and they need special care and protection.

All in all, I feel that most birds with damaged beaks may experience future growth abnormalities and should never be released.

Abnormal beaks. Some birds do manage to survive in the wild with mis-shapen beaks but eventually they are unable to feed, become weak and, if they are lucky, are picked up. More often than not, the beaks are overgrown and need filing back into shape. A set of half-round small files or one of the model-makers' electric drills with a selection of mini grinding bits are ideal for the purpose. The beak may bleed if it is cut too short but a dab with a caustic pencil should stop any serious blood loss.

Once again, remember that crossbills naturally have crossed mandibles for opening their pine-cone food.

Bleeding (see Skin Wounds, Ch. 3, pp. 70–2)

Cloacitis (constipation)
A healthy bird's droppings are made up of two components – the dark

portion being any solid waste, with the white portion being the urates excreted by the kidneys. If a bird cannot stand for any length of time, then its cloaca can be impeded and it becomes unable to excrete any waste material. Then a large calculus of urates will build up inside the body, blocking any passage of faeces. This build-up can be felt as a hard lump just forward of the cloaca where the bird's abdominal area is usually soft.

Syringing liquid paraffin well into the cloaca will help the bird expel the calculus, which will also be softened and broken up by the liquid paraffin. Remember that the cloaca has a degree of elasticity which will help you remove any lumps. Just make sure that the bird is not suffering from egg-binding (see p. 51) because fracture of the egg would cause all sorts of problems.

Concussion

Concussion is one of the most common injuries to wild birds. Typically caused by collisions with cars or windows, symptoms can include the loss of use of the legs, loss of balance and an inability to hold the head upright. In fact, sometimes the head is held upside down. One method I use to confirm concussion is to look directly along the bird's beak at both eyes, making sure, of course, that it cannot peck my face. Both eyes should appear identical: if one is slightly more closed than the other, concussion is likely. However, do not be fooled by an infected or damaged eye (see p. 52–3).

There are no sophisticated treatments, like brain scans and lengthy steroid courses, as there are for humans. Usually warmth and semi-darkness with supportive fluid therapy (see Ch. 1, pp. 35–40) is all that can be done. If the concussion continues for some days, force-feeding may be necessary.

More intense initial treatment can be given under the auspices of a vet, who can prescribe one or two doses of dexamethasone, injected subcutaneously or intramuscularly.

If there is no improvement after a few days, then the damage to the brain is probably not going to get any better, although the bird may cope in captivity. On the other hand, we did have a redwing with a damaged eye that was causing infection to the brain and a typical upturned head. Treatment was with chloromycetin succinate and what had seemed a hopeless case is now behaving normally. (This treatment was very sophisticated and suggested by our specialist veterinary consultant as there was the faint hope of a cure.)

Crop problems

Apart from the common injury of a ruptured crop, dealt with in the chapter on skin wounds (Ch. 3, pp. 75–6), most crop problems occur as a direct result of bad feeding. Always feel a bird's crop to see if it is full of unsuitable food that has remained undigested. This can then be squeezed back up the throat and out through the mouth. A few millilitres of liquid paraffin gavaged (see Ch. 1, pp. 38–40) into the crop will help any residues pass through. Incidents I have seen include a swan that gorged itself and blocked its crop with corn; great crested grebes blocking their crops with feathers swallowed while preening; a robin full of uncooked dough and numerous pigeons chock-a-block with enormous acorns.

Hard unmoving lumps may be lesions of trichomoniasis (see pp. 66–8).

Dislocations (see Ch. 3, pp. 88–90)

Ear problems

A bird's ears are very similar in function to those of mammals, except they do not have the exterior trumpets for sound collection. Situated more or less behind the eyes, they can be seen as spotlessly clean holes when the small head feathers covering them are gently parted. Owls' ears are different from other birds' in that each is set at a different level to make locating the sound and position of their prey possible on the darkest night. The 'long ears' and 'short ears' of long- and short-eared owls are, in fact, feather tufts on top of their heads; their actual ears are in the same position as those of other owls.

Birds generally have few problems with ear infections, but if, on examination, the ear holes seem clogged or have a discharge, then your vet might like to prescribe Panalog Ointment (Ciba-Geigy) to squeeze into the ear sockets.

Head injuries and damage to the skull may present some bleeding from the ears. Only rest and treatment for concussion (see above) can help the bird recover. Damage to the delicate balance mechanism of the inner ear may result in head tilts or lack of co-ordination in standing. As with all other head injuries, it is a question of 'wait and see' if the bird gets better.

Similar loss-of-balance symptoms without a history of trauma may indicate an inner ear infection which needs treatment with systemic antibiotics (see Ch. 3, pp. 76–8). In this situation we would administer long-acting amoxycillin, available from a vet, daily for at least five days.

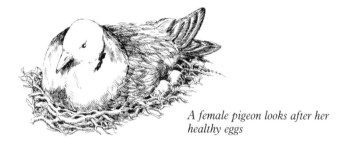

A female pigeon looks after her healthy eggs

Egg binding

Egg binding is usually caused either by a normal or even an over-large egg being trapped in the oviduct by spasms of the muscles or, the opposite, failure of the muscles to expel the egg. The egg can be clearly felt in the soft abdomen just forward of the cloaca (anus). It is crucial not to break the egg, which can usually be worked out of an anaesthetised bird, especially if a little liquid paraffin is syringed into the cloaca. Anaesthetics in birds is little understood in the veterinary world, but we have found Isoflurane (Abbott Laboratories) to be safer than most. An old wives' tail of steaming the bird over a hot kettle is unlikely to bring relief. However, an injection of Oxytocin and calcium by the vet may stimulate the bird to pass the egg.

Endoparasites

Most wild birds have some type of internal parasite load. In most cases the bird and its worms live in harmony. Parasites, however, can cause problems and are best dealt with as a matter of routine in every bird that is handled. The current thinking is that a broad-spectrum anthelmintic (wormer) like ivermectin (Ivomec-MSD Agvet) given orally or by subcutaneous injection will clear most, including the syngamus gapeworms (see below).

Eye problems

By far the most important sense to a wild bird is its sight. Birds, except perhaps vultures, have little or no sense of smell and rely on their sight to feed, even in captivity. There are, though, one or two exceptions, notably the captive owl that could feel with the vibrissae (whiskers) around its beak, and a recent woodcock casualty that felt for its food with the sensitive tip of its very long bill.

Most birds can survive with one eye, but even with monocular vision the daytime hunters, like hawks and falcons, cannot catch prey and should not be released. Owls can use their ears for locating prey when hunting and many one-eyed owls manage well in the wild. Nevertheless, the treatment and care of eyes is of the utmost importance.

We all know how sensitive our own eyes can be. Birds are no different and I would recommend nothing more than rinsing or bathing a bird's eye with clean warm water, using a cotton bud or cotton wool. Even if the lids are stuck together, use the warm water – do not be tempted by proprietary eye washes.

Quite unlike humans, birds have a third eyelid, the nictitating membrane, under the outer lids. This constantly slides across the eyeball, providing it with essential moisture and cleaning any dust or debris away. If for any reason a bird cannot close or cover an eye, then there is a likelihood that the eye will suffer permanent damage because it will dry out. Hypromellose drops, available from a vet, applied several times daily will keep the eye moist, but far less time consuming is the application of the ointment Lacri-Lube (Allergan), available from chemists. Either preparation can be used to keep the eye moist until specialist veterinary attention can be found.

Never put any other preparations into an eye, especially not those containing corticosteroids, unless you are advised by a specialist veterinary surgeon. A safe antibiotic lubricant for eye infections is plain chloramphenicol eye ointment, available from a vet, which should be applied to the lower lid several times daily to be of any use.

Sometimes a bird's eye can be affected by **mites**, which are seen as moving specks of dust around an inflamed eye. A very mild insect powder, Rid-Mite (Johnsons), available from pet shops, will clear them after one or two daily dustings.

Vitamin deficiencies can and will cause eye problems but if every wild bird in care is given a vitamin supplement in its feed, the problem should never arise.

Eye problems can signify more deep-seated infections and if you take in a collared dove or other pigeon with an obvious problem in just one eye, then keep it separate from all other birds and handle it only with rubber gloves. The bird could be harbouring a disease infectious to other birds or could, just possibly, be suffering from ornithosis, the non-parrot form of psittacosis, which is still contagious to humans. If in any doubt, have the bird checked by a veterinary practice which will, if the tests prove positive, advise that the bird be destroyed. Although not as virulent as parrot-borne psittacosis, it can still be lethal to humans and can be breathed in even after the bird itself is cured.

After even a suspected case, thoroughly wash and sterilise in parvocide, available from pet stores, everything the bird has been in contact with. Do not panic, though, for I have taken in and treated many thousands of wild birds and have only seen ornithosis on one occasion, in a run of infected collared doves, but it always pays to be on the lookout and very meticulous with hygiene in the handling of birds.

Feather damage

A bird's feathers give it a highly adjustable protective coat against all weather conditions, as well as providing the aerodynamics necessary for flight and manoeuvre. Any damage, even to a single feather, could jeopardise these abilities, exposing the bird to cold, wet and starvation. Hawks and falcons are particularly susceptible to the latter as the loss of only one wing or tail feather could hinder their hunting ability.

Feathers are like hair, growing out of follicles in the skin and being replaced regularly during the moult. New feathers are called 'pin' feathers and may get broken in accidents, resulting in a surprising amount of bleeding. Birds do not have a lot of blood, so it is essential that any bleeding feathers are clamped off with artery forceps or else tied off with cotton. Fortunately, a bird's blood clots easily and after a few minutes the bleeding should have stopped.

A **broken feather** will not grow again and will only be replaced at the next moult, which could be a year away. Plucking the feather will encourage a replacement to grow but may cause damage to the follicle, so I only recommend it if there is no alternative.

Pigeons and doves, however, have the ability to lose their feathers at the slightest hint of a tug. It's probably a good way of leaving a predator with a mouthful of feathers but it's frustrating when you are trying to catch a dove and end up with only its tail in your hand. The tail will soon regrow, but you have probably lost your bird.

The only time when plucking feathers is necessary is when you need to clean and treat a skin wound. In the main, the feathers around a wound are only small down feathers and these come out with a short, sharp tug. Artery forceps are very useful for pulling out stubborn feathers, including the occasional large primary (on the outside of the wing) or secondary feathers (on the inner part of the wing) that may be aggravating a wing wound.

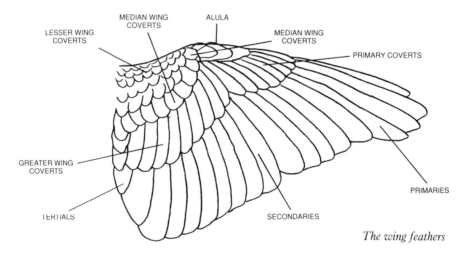

The wing feathers

A broken feather is not a major problem to a pigeon or a thrush but it could mean life or death to specialist fliers like swifts or kestrels.

Swift feathers often get damaged and dishevelled by untimely landings on the ground. Before any grounded swift is launched back to its aerial existence (see Ch. 1, p. 13) it can have any damaged feathers *haute coutured* over a steaming kettle just by holding the damaged feathers in the jet of steam and slowly stroking the feathers back into shape.

Bent or creased feathers on a larger bird can be straightened and then held rigid with a dab of glue from a DIY hot-glue gun across the inevitable crease.

A falconry method of repairing feathers of a bird of prey is called 'imping'. A piece of feather, similar to the broken feather, is cut to the same size as the broken or missing portion. As feathers are hollow, a thin stick covered in glue is passed into the stub of feather on the bird, while a new piece is slid over the stick to join up as one. It's worthwhile adopting this system for the tails of woodpeckers, as these birds use them as supports while they are on the trunks of trees.

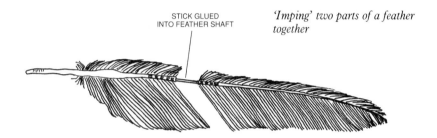

STICK GLUED
INTO FEATHER SHAFT

'Imping' two parts of a feather together

Feather lice are part of the normal parasite load of all wild birds, especially swans. They do not normally cause any problems, whereas feather mites, the other common ectoparasite, seen as moving dust particles, can weaken feathers. If necessary both can be controlled with Rid-Mite powder, available from pet shops.

Light coloured bars across the feathers are fret marks caused by a shortage of food during the growth of a new feather. They are not usually a problem but can be a site of weakness for the stronger, flying birds of prey. If in doubt, a dab with the hot-glue gun will add strength.

Oil on feathers (see Ch. 4, pp. 92–5)

Foot problems
In my experience, a bird's foot is the most tender part of its body and is normally well protected in the wild. Casualties seem to experience very little trouble with their feet, except those snared in cotton or fishing line (see Ch. 4, p. 91). In captivity, however, many species are susceptible to foot problems and vulnerable species like birds of prey and water birds should be monitored closely.

A well-known term in the captive-bird world is **bumblefoot**, a persistent infection causing pain and swelling mainly on the ball of the foot. Apart from swans, where bumblefoot appears to be routine, I have only once seen the infection in a wild bird – a little owl – although I did take in a green woodpecker with gout, which produced similar lesions. It should not occur in wild birds but is likely to affect any bird kept in captivity for any length of time. It is a stubborn infection to treat, so preventative measures, such as providing natural perches from the outset, will save you from a host of problems later in a bird's stay with you.

EXPERIENCE HAS SHOWN THAT FOOT PROBLEMS IN BIRDS IN CAPTIVITY, HOUSED BOTH IN CAGES AND IN AVIARIES, CAN BE AVOIDED BY USING A SELECTION OF SIZES OF BRANCHES AS NATURAL PERCHES, RATHER THAN THE SMOOTH WOODEN TYPES SO POPULAR (WRONGLY SO) IN THE CAGES OF BUDGIES AND CANARIES.

Apart from bumblefoot in water birds, and it does not seem to hamper them, the most susceptible species are birds of prey. Initial causes can be when a rear toe talon punctures the ball of the foot, or when the bird can only use one leg and is forced to put all its weight on it. Perches padded with carpet will help prevent a disabled bird of prey developing a problem in what may be its only good foot.

If there is any suspicion of bumblefoot in a bird of prey, the bird should be referred to an experienced avian veterinarian, who can take samples of the infection and advise on suitable antibiotic therapy or remedial surgery.

Except for birds of prey, swans and woodpeckers, most birds seem to be able to manage on one foot. But if there is any doubt about a bird coping with this disability, it should not be released. Woodpeckers and birds of prey can flourish in captivity on one foot, but swans will probably have to be destroyed unless an innovative prosthesis can be designed.

Water birds in captivity often suffer from foot conditions, especially if they have to be denied access to water. Their feet and the webbing may dry and crack, causing them to limp. Regular applications of cod liver oil ointment or E45 cream will help to alleviate any discomfort.

A bird may sometimes be presented to you with **one or both feet tightly clenched** in paralysis. A single foot clenched like this may just be the result of trauma or a sprain and can be exercised by stretching the

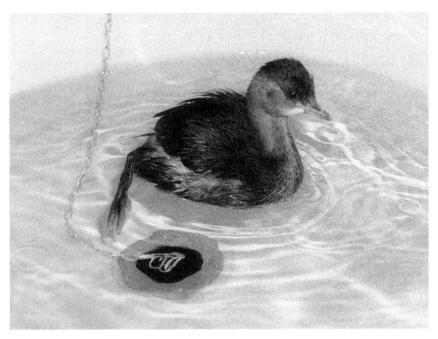

A water bird's feet can suffer in captivity if it does not have access to water

leg, making the toes flex and unflex. Spasms in both feet can also be the result of trauma but are more likely to suggest some other cause, like poisoning (see Ch. 4, pp. 96–8). Similar physiotherapy may help but there are likely to be other spasms in various parts of the body, especially in the wings, and sedation with a valium injection will bring relief to the bird. Once again, an avian veterinarian will advise if further treatments may be necessary.

Force-feeding

A bird can be safely rehydrated by gavaging with fluids, but fluids contain no nourishment so after just a short time, six hours in the case of small birds, more substantial support is needed. Liquid foods like Complan, Ensure and Liquivite are all suitable as initial substitutes, but should be supplemented with a more natural solid diet as soon as possible. Liquid foods can, of course, be gavaged, but the more solid diets may need to be force-fed.

Force-feeding should be regarded as a drastic course of action, a last resort to be used if your bird is not feeding itself after just a short time in captivity. Really tiny birds like wrens and goldcrests will not last long without feeding and are really too small to stand the manhandling of forcing food into them. The only solution with birds of that size is to try to tempt them with tasty morsels of live food like greenfly, fruit fly or tiny spiders, their favourite. Other birds should not be fed immediately on arrival – you should wait until any fluid therapy (see Ch. 1, pp. 35–40) has stabilised their condition and then offer them their natural food, whether it be seed, insects or fish.

Birds may not feed because of weakness or because they have specialised feeding habits and cannot cope with the food as we present it. A typical example is the swift, a bird which trawls for insects while high in the sky and does not have the ability to peck food off the ground or out of a dish. Other birds, like kingfishers, grebes and auks, may have to be force-fed with fish for the first day or two, but should then start helping themselves out of a dish. To force-feed a bird with fish, hold the bird's beak open then slide the whole fish – whitebait, sprats or small herrings – headfirst down the throat until the bird swallows because of its own reflexes. All fish should be fresh or freshly defrosted, wet and still cold, or the bird may reject it.

Birds reluctant to feed may just copy one of their own species – a good case for keeping unreleasable birds as therapy for the new casualties.

Most force-feeding is carried out using liquid diets like Complan or Ensure, gavaged in the same way as for fluid therapy. Swifts can be force-fed by gavaging 'St Tiggywinkles glop' straight into their crops once or twice a day using a 1ml syringe.

Recipe for St Tiggywinkles Glop

1 tin Pedigree Chum puppy food
1 tin dried insects (Sluis Universal Food or Prosecto)
1 tin water
1 pinch high-calorie vitamin supplement
1 pinch bone meal supplement
1 pinch Can-addase enzyme supplement

Liquidise everything to the consistency of soft ice cream and replace after 24 hours.

Owls, **hawks** and **kestrels** have to be force-fed with whole or chopped mice, which are available frozen via advertisements in the weekly paper *Cage and Aviary Birds*.

A typical forced diet for an adult swan would be:
one whole packet of Complan
half packet of Lectade
1.7l warm water
gavaged at 180ml per day

Head damage (see also Concussion, above)
It has now been proved that birds which collide with windows suffer most commonly not from a broken neck but, to some degree, from cerebral haemorrhage. The apparent broken neck is merely a flaccid paralysis noticeable in an unconscious bird or one that has recently died. Treatment should be for concussion, there is nothing else that can be done except to make the bird as comfortable and quiet as possible.

Place the bird in a warm, dark, quiet box with an old towel to stand on and wait for it to recover. Never leave it with a water dish just in case it falls into it. Occasionally, say every half an hour, dip the bird's beak in a bowl of Lectade or rehydrating fluid (see Ch. 1, p. 29).

Quite often a bird will be found with most of the skin torn from its head, exposing the skull. This is often the result of skirmishes with other birds. As long as the skull and brain are not damaged the bird should cope, although it may always be bald. Treat the area just like any other skin wound (see under Abrasions, p. 47).

Fractures (see Ch. 1, pp. 32–5 and Ch. 3, pp. 79–88)

Hyperthermia
As opposed to the well-known human condition, hypothermia, hyperthermia is caused by overheating or heatstroke and is not uncommon in birds.

Birds have no means of disposing of excess heat through their skin other than by fluffing out their feathers to allow cooler air to circulate. Their main means of cooling themselves is to open their beaks and pant. Owls, in particular, will palpate their throats to disperse body heat created, particularly, by stress.

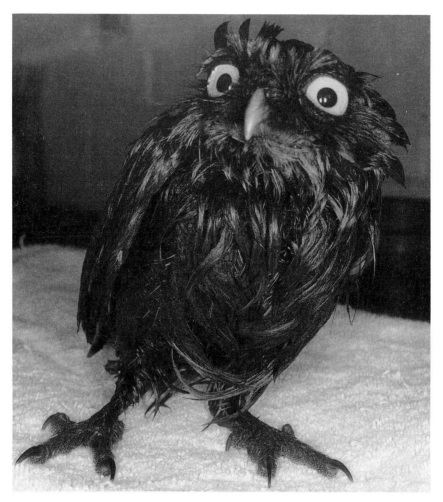

Hypothermia can set in if the waterproof feathers are contaminated with oil

The common occurrences of hyperthermia are in unfeathered hatchlings exposed to strong sunlight, or in birds kept in unsuitable or incorrectly controlled heated containers. In any case, the bird will need to be moved to a cooler situation and fluids given by gavage (see Ch. 1, pp. 38–40) or subcutaneously (see Ch. 3, pp. 76–7). If the bird is obviously in dire straits, then a dunking in cold water will help cool it and ease the condition.

Hypothermia

Although this is a fairly common condition in elderly humans, its full implications and the damage it can cause are still not completely understood. Birds can usually cope with intensely cold conditions as long as they are able to find food and can keep dry. Any breakdown of their waterproof feather mantle with oil or other contaminant allows rain or water to percolate through to the skin, very quickly chilling them – the first stage of hypothermia.

During hypothermia, just as in shock, the bird's circulatory system closes off outlying blood vessels and capillaries, making the bird's skin feel cold to the touch. As a result of the loss of blood supply to these outer areas, there is no removal of cellular waste products, leading to progressive cell deaths until the bird itself dies. A bird with obvious hypothermia will feel cold and lifeless. The priority is to get those closed blood vessels opened again and the circulation back in full flow. The immediate treatment can be to dunk your bird in a bowl of very warm water – but do be careful as it may well chill again once it is removed.

Fluids will help restore the circulation but do need to be warmed before administration either by gavage (see Ch. 1, pp. 38–40) or preferably intravenously in boluses small enough not to damage the blood vessels. Leaving a catheter inserted in a vein saves you having to keep re-entering the fragile venous systems. Dexamethasone will also help to open closed peripheral blood vessels.

This emergency treatment obviously needs the expertise of someone used to working on birds. But don't give up if there isn't anyone of that description around – many hypothermic birds will still recover on their own, provided they are warmed through. When they show signs of recovery, which can be fairly rapid, offer a drink of Lectade or rehydrating fluid (see Ch. 1, p. 29) and withhold food for at least 12 hours to give the circulatory system time to adjust from the trauma.

Internal parasites (see Endoparasites, p. 51)

Leeches

Many water birds, notably swans, ducks and gulls, are being adversely affected by masses of leeches on their heads; in their eyes, mouths, nostrils and upper respiratory tract. You do not need to dab each one with a cigarette, as Humphrey Bogart did in *The African Queen*, but they do need to be removed.

Dunking the bird's whole head in a bucket of cold, clean water for 10 seconds may dislodge most. Any remaining, especially in the eyes and deep in the nostrils, will have to be picked off with forceps or tweezers. Plain chloramphenicol eye ointment, applied just once, will cure any soreness in the eyes.

Leg fractures (see Ch. 3, pp. 79–82)

Lice (see Feather damage, p. 55)

Ligatures (see skin wounds and their treatment, Ch. 3, pp. 70–5)

Maggots

During the warmer months any wound is in danger of becoming 'fly blown', that is, infected with maggots. There is no easy way to kill these off and remove them, other than by painstakingly picking them off one by one with forceps or tweezers and cleaning the wound site with dilute Savlon or Hibiscrub (see Ch. 2, p. 47). Look under the wings at the shoulder and under the legs at the hips.

Massive wounds can be packed with Battle's Fly and Maggot Paste.

Maggots dislike hot, dry conditions so some success can be achieved by drying the area with an electric hair drier, but be careful not to burn the bird. Covering the birds head will keep it calm.

EVERY SINGLE MAGGOT HAS TO BE REMOVED OR ELSE THE BIRD WILL BE KILLED OR SO SEVERELY INJURED THAT IT HAS NO FUTURE.

Mites (see Feather damage, p. 55)

Respiratory infection

Birds have a totally different system of breathing from our own and that of other mammals. In order to service their high metabolic rate and the immense energy required for flying, they have not only rudimentary lungs but also a system of air-sacs, which even include hollow bones (humeri) in their wings as part of the network. In fact, in one of those atrocious nineteenth-century animal experiments, a scientist proved that a strangled chicken could still breathe through a broken wing.

Instead of the simple in-and-out muscular breathing of a mammal, a bird's intake of air is caused by the air of the previous breath passing from the lungs into the air-sacs. So, before being expired at the next breath, as a bird breathes its chest deflates and then fills with fresh air by vacuum action, whereas a mammal's chest fills and then empties by the action of the rib muscles. Because of this, birds under gaseous anaesthetic can have gas trapped in their air-sacs even after the anaesthetic is turned off. THIS CALLS FOR THE USE OF ONLY SAFE ANAESTHETICS IN BIRDS, WHICH AT THE MOMENT SEEMS TO BE ISOFLURANE, ADMINISTERED BY A SHORTENED PAEDIATRIC ENDOTRACHEAL TUBE. DO NOT LET YOUR BIRDS BE ANAESTHETISED WITH ANY OTHER INHALATION AGENT AS THEY WILL PROBABLY DIE.

Because of the lack of a really noticeable rise and fall of a bird's chest, the way to diagnose a respiratory infection is to see if the bird breathes with its mouth open. That is, unless it is under stress or overheating with hyperthermia. Except for some birds like the gannet, the inhalation of air starts at the nares, or nostrils – two holes situated at the top of the beak. These can easily become clogged, especially those of baby birds that are being fed by hand. Bathing with a weak saline solution, with cotton wool or a cotton bud, and the careful removal of any debris will soon clear them. (A weak saline solution is 0.9% table salt, dissolved in distilled water.)

Leeches can cause blockages in the nares of water birds, as can the contusions caused by the scaly face-mite, *Cnemidocoptes pilae*. These can usually be seen under a magnifying glass and then loosened with a drop of liquid paraffin. Ivermectin (Ivomec-MSD Agvet) may be useful in clearing the complete infestation.

An apparently **runny nose** can indicate an upper respiratory tract infection that may need antibiotics to clear it up. **Sinusitis** in birds is far more serious than in humans, with the sinuses around the eyes and forehead becoming swollen and blocked with infection. It is serious because surgery may be required to clear any infection which, in a bird, is usually seen as a solid, cheese-like pus.

Further on down the respiratory tract, inhaled air passes through the roof of the mouth (the choanae), from where it passes through the glottis down into the trachea (the airway leading to the lungs).

The glottis is situated immediately behind the tongue. It is constantly opening and closing as the bird breathes and should appear pink and flexible. Fluid passing through the glottis into the trachea and then to the lungs, and lesions of trichomoniasis (see pp. 66–8) partially blocking it, are the two major concerns.

Syngamus, the gape worms, can sometimes be spotted just inside the glottis attached to the wall of the trachea. Treatment is the same as for other internal parasites – ivermectin (available from a vet or pharmaceutical merchant).

The main body of the respiratory system, the trachea, lungs and air-sacs are particularly susceptible to **fungus invasion** either by aspergillus or candida spores. **Aspergillosis** is likely to flare up in any captive wild bird, especially those with air-sac damage. Sea birds like **divers** and **auks** appear to fail through aspergillosis rather than any other problem. All our sea birds intake is now routinely dosed with ketoconazole (Nizoral-Janssen) or miconazole (Daktarin-Janssen) to counter the inevitable fungal invasion. Nizoral is available from vets, Daktarin from chemists. It's nigh on impossible to assess whether or not a bird has aspergillosis but if in any doubt either of these oral preparations will help.

The air-sacs themselves are often punctured, especially by cats, resulting sometimes in swellings under the skin (subcutaneous emphysema). It's not possible to perform heroic suturing on torn air-sacs but most will heal spontaneously if they are re-covered with the surrounding skin and the bird treated with antibiotics and anti-fungals. Antibiotics and Nizoral must be prescribed by a vet who will give directions on use. Daktarin is an oral gel available from chemists and is given by mouth daily at 0.5ml per 250g.

Ruptured crop (see under Skin Wounds, Ch. 3, pp. 75–6)

Septicaemia

Septicaemia is the term for the presence in the bloodstream of potentially fatal pathogenic bacteria. Once it gets a hold it is very difficult to shift and prevention is better than attempting a cure, which, in spite of antibiotics, may not always be successful.

Cat bites. Until recently, nearly every bird caught by a cat died within 48 hours. The inevitable demise was put down to shock and was accepted as that. However, it has recently been proved that most of the deaths are due to septicaemia infection introduced by the bacteria, *Pasteurella multicoda*, found on a cat's teeth.

To counter this we now routinely inject every bird suspected of being caught by a cat with one dose of long-acting amoxycillin antibiotic. Once started, a course of antibiotics should normally be completed, but we found that the added stress of further handling and subsequent injections did more harm than good and the one injection has improved our success rate to nearly 100%, provided the injuries are not too severe.

It is normally routine to weigh a bird before administering drugs but to save the stress of unnecessary handling, we have **standard doses of long-acting amoxycillin** for different sized birds. These are:
sparrow-sized birds 0.05ml
blackbird-sized birds 0.10ml
collared dove-sized birds 0.25ml
pigeon-sized birds 0.5ml

Shot wounds (see Ch. 3, pp. 78–9)

Skin wounds (see Ch. 3, pp. 70–2)

Starvation (see Fluid therapy, Ch. 1, pp. 35–40; Force-feeding, pp. 57–9, and Hypothermia, p. 61)

Stress
All wild birds taken into captivity are going to be under some degree of stress. Handling should always be kept to a minimum and if possible never look directly at the bird unless a specific treatment is being given. Also, birds are not used to looking up to people so, ideally, any cages should be placed over two metres from the ground.

Some birds seem to be particularly vulnerable to stress and will die at the drop of a hat. The species that spring to mind are **sparrowhawks**, **ospreys** and, surprisingly enough, **pheasants**. Whenever we take in one of these three 'scatty' species we cover the cage with a light cloth for at least two days before we will even contemplate assessing their injuries, unless these are bleeding wounds, compound fractures or similar conditions that demand urgent stabilisation.

Treatment with diazepam (from a vet) can be particularly effective and safe for birds which refuse to settle.

IN GENERAL, IF ANY BIRD YOU ARE HANDLING STARTS TO GASP AND BREATHE THROUGH ITS MOUTH, THEN PUT IT BACK IMMEDIATELY INTO A WARM CAGE AND DO NOT PICK IT UP AGAIN FOR ONE OR TWO HOURS. IT WILL DIE IN SECONDS IF YOU KEEP HOLDING IT.

Subcutaneous emphysema

Often a bird will come in with one or even numerous transparent swellings on its body. These are the result of punctures of the air-sacs, which have allowed air to collect under the skin and stretch it just like a balloon.

These swellings around the neck and other joints can severely impair movement, often making it impossible for the bird to stand up. To relieve them, swab the area with dilute Savlon, Hibiscrub (see Ch. 2, p. 47) or surgical spirit – use the last only on unbroken skin – and pierce the swelling with a sterile needle, gently squeezing to expel the air. The damaged air-sac should heal spontaneously but in the meantime the swellings may re-appear and again need lancing.

Syngamus (Gape Worm) (see Endoparasites, p. 51)

Tongue

A bird's tongue is easily visible as an arrow shape lying in the bottom of the beak. The usual injuries include fishing line or cotton wrapped around the base, although we did have to stitch back on a duck's tongue, which had been nearly severed by the plastic rings off a four-pack of beer.

Most birds can survive with a damaged tongue or even without one altogether. Woodpeckers, though, use their extra-long tongues for feeding and may have great problems if theirs do not heal perfectly.

Trichomoniasis

Known as 'trick' to wild bird rehabilitators, canker to pigeon fanciers and frounce to falconers, this is a common ailment, particularly in pigeons and doves and, unlike other internal parasites, this one will definitely kill the bird. The villains are trichomonads, minute swimming animals, the product of which forms a cheese-like growth in the back of the mouth, throat and crop. Death is caused by starvation as the growth blocks the throat, or by suffocation or drowning if it invades the glottis.

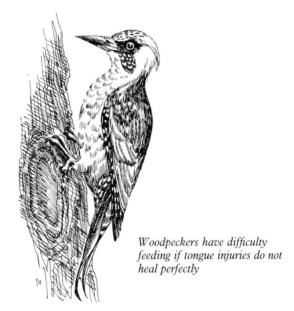

Woodpeckers have difficulty feeding if tongue injuries do not heal perfectly

Opening an infected bird's beak will usually reveal the cheese-like mass, which will be accompanied by a typically foul smell. Sometimes the lesions are on the crop and cannot be seen, but they can be felt as a hard, unmoving lump. Wherever they are, do not be tempted to chip away at the cheesy masses as they may be eroding some of the major blood vessels. It is possible to pass a gavage tube (see Ch. 1, pp. 38–40) past the mass to administer fluids to counter the inevitable starvation. A very slight dash of Hibiscrub in the fluids will help clean any infected areas.

Treatment is with tablets of Spartrix (Janssen), administered with a plastic pill-giver. An oral administration by gavage tube of metronidazole can also be effective. Both these drugs can be obtained from a vet, although Spartrix may be available at some pharmacies.

After a few days the mass should start to break away by itself and a little cooking oil can be rubbed into it to help soften it up so the bird can start feeding again. Most birds can manage to drink Lectade after their initial treatment of fluids.

Vitamin deficiency

Birds tend to be more susceptible to vitamin deficiencies than mammals and bird casualties, or birds in captivity should have a multi-vitamin supplement added to all their feed. Live food like maggots or meal-worms should always be sprinkled with vitamin powder. Most wild birds manage to maintain their own vitamin balances but occasionally, particularly in water birds, vitamin deficiencies can be observed.

Vitamin A deficiency may show as discharges from the mouth, eyes, nares and cloaca. If in doubt give one of the vitamin A pills available from pet shops.

Vitamin B1 this is the vitamin thiamine that is destroyed by a white fish diet. Supplement B1 vitamins should be given as a matter of course to any bird on such a diet. Symptoms of a deficiency include lethargy, a loss of appetite, a loss of balance and contraction of the pupils.

Vitamin B Complex deficiency may cause leg and wing weakness as well as poor feathering and muscle disorders.

Vitamin D is the vitamin of bone building and a shortage may lead to rickets in a growing bird. Sterile bone meal added to the feed of young birds should prevent it happening to any in your care.

Vitamin E deficiency shows itself as a wastage of muscle fibres causing, amongst other symptoms, standing difficulties. Wheatgerm and green vegetables are a safe way of restoring the balance.

It seems to me that, apart from vitamin B1 deficiency, which can be diagnosed conclusively, most vitamin deficiency diagnoses are very vague. Except in instances of vitamin B1 shortage, therefore, a general multivitamin like Abidec, SA37 or Vet-a-min are entirely suitable, with an injection of B complex vitamins (Parentrovite) or B12 as a quick tonic for a weak new casualty.

Weakness

By weakness I mean an inability to stand or fly, which can be assessed by feeling the general condition of the bird. A weak bird with good, solid muscle on both sides of its keel (breast bone) will have been feeding up until recently, so its problems have been very short-lived. Likely diagnoses could be trauma, concussion or poisoning.

A bird that is both weak and very thin has been suffering for some while and has been unable or unwilling to feed. Things to look for are disease, internal or external parasites, damage to its beak, or eyes, blockage of the oesophagus by fishing line; or could the emaciation be caused by a long spell of extreme cold or dry weather? In addition to treating the cause of the weakness, fluid therapy (see Ch. 1, pp. 35–40) and liquid nutrition will help the bird regain its strength.

Wing fractures (see Ch. 3, pp. 83–5)

Worms (see Endoparasites, p. 51)

This chapter contains the one-off individual situations that crop up occasionally. In the following chapters I will describe the conditions that occur among most casualties that are taken into care, in particular skin wounds and fractures, and their treatment.

3

Skin Wounds and Fractures

Their maintenance and care, including gunshot wounds and suturing

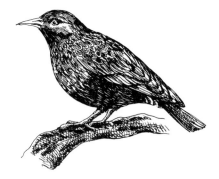

SKIN WOUNDS

Any wild bird casualty taken into care should be thoroughly examined for skin wounds. These can range from minor pecks on the head or simple grazes, to massive skin losses, particularly when an owl gets itself caught on a barbed wire fence. Gunshot wounds are, unfortunately, very common and can usually be identified as such. Wounds on the rump, around the preen gland, although mysterious are almost invariably caused by a cat bite. Fishing line and cotton cause cutting wounds, particularly to the legs and feet, which sometimes need suturing, if only to keep the leg or foot in shape.

NEVER TAKE IT FOR GRANTED THAT THE WOUND YOU HAVE FOUND IS THE ONLY ONE. CHECK EVERY INCH OF THE BIRD LOOKING FOR THE TELL-TALE SIGNS OF MATTED FEATHERS, SOMETIMES WITH BLOOD STAINS. Luckily, a bird's blood clots quite quickly and it is unlikely that a live bird will be found that is still bleeding. The exceptions, however, are those suffering from broken feathers or talons, both of which conditions may continue to bleed profusely until you intervene.

Finding and cleaning

Once any wounds have been located, place the bird on a heated mat or a hot water bottle covered with an old towel. Covering its head will keep the bird quiet while you treat the wounds. Even under cover some birds are still dangerous so take precautions before you start or else I guarantee you will get bitten or 'footed', the falconry term.

Precautions when handling different species could be:

Hawks, falcons, owls – temporarily tape the feet together with zinc oxide plaster

Crows, rooks and other Corvids – wrap an elastic band around beaks to stop them biting

Herons, gannets, cormorants, hawks – should be held by another person while you work

Grebes and divers – heads should be covered by towels taped in place

Swans – will not bite but their wings should be controlled by another person

Most other species, even if they do bite, can do little damage, making it unnecessary to take specific precautions. In order to clean any wounds properly the wound must be totally exposed, even though this involves plucking any feathers from around the wound site. Most of the lesser feathers – the down feathers – will come away quite easily, the larger ones may need a quick sharp tug, but do be careful not to tear the skin even more. It's not a good idea to try plucking the primary flight feathers, as the effort needed may cause permanent damage to the feather follicles. Any of these feathers in the way of a wound can be cut as short as possible with sharp scissors. Bleeding of these feathers should be stemmed by clamping them with artery forceps or dabbing with a caustic pencil.

Clean the wounds with a dilute solution of either Savlon or Hibiscrub (see Ch. 2, p. 47) warmed to body temperature. Cotton wool balls are ideal as swabs. The wound should be thoroughly washed from the centre outwards. Cotton buds are useful for cleaning small wounds, with a pair of clean forceps handy to remove any feathers or other debris from the wound site. A nozzle or Spreull's needle fitted to a 20ml syringe allows you to squirt dilute Savlon or Hibiscrub into the wound to flush out any unseen debris.

A light application of Scherisorb gel (Smith and Nephew), available at chemists, will help the wound heal and in most cases nothing else needs to be done. As long as your cleaning regime was thorough, the bird's natural resistance to infection will allow the wound to heal within a few days.

WOUNDS THAT NEED SUTURING

Some wounds, however, will never heal on their own, either because there is considerable damage, or because there is an infection. For a wound on a bird to heal, the edges of that wound need to be touching, or, if there is some skin loss, there should be no movement of the skin over the underlying tissues. If the casualty has a deep wound or if the skin has been torn from the tissue base, then the wound may need suturing. I am sure your vet will advise on your first few cases that need suturing and he or she will probably instruct you on techniques and materials to use so that you do not have to keep interrupting the busy veterinary practices for minor skin wounds.

BIRDS REGISTER NO DISCOMFORT WHILE HAVING WOUNDS SUTURED AND VERY SELDOM NEED ANAESTHETISING. LOCAL ANAESTHETIC –

Absorbable Suturing Materials

Catgut
Polyglycolic acid (Dexon)
Polyglactin 910 (Vicryl)
Polydioxanone (PDS)

Non-absorbable Suturing Materials

Silk
Nylon and cotton
Polypropylene (Prolene)
Polymerized caprolactam (Supramid, Vetafil)
Polyesters (Dacron, Mersilene, Ethiboud)

ANALGESICS – ARE NOT RECOMMENDED FOR USE IN BIRDS, WHO MAY REACT STRONGLY AGAINST THEM.

Various materials are available for suturing, composed either of absorbable or non-absorbable material, the latter having to be removed at a later date, normally seven days. Absorbable sutures are used for stitching up internal damage, such as on muscles and tendons. Examples are shown in the box on the previous page.

Most of these come in small sterile packs already attached to needles of various sizes. These are the preferred types for use in birds as they are much narrower than eyed needles and do less damage to the fragile skin. A good, cheap or even free source of them is your local hospital where, once the outer wrapping has been opened, the still-sealed pack is discarded if not used. The packets have a life-size diagram of the enclosed needle on the outside but the thickness of the suture may be confusing. Two sizes are shown, both meaning the same thickness but using different descriptions. For instance:

Suture size	
Metric (actual size ×10)	USP
1	5.0
1.5	4.0 thin
2	3.0 through
3	2.0 to
3.5	0 thick
4	1
5	2

Added advantages of these packaged sutures is that they retain their sterility until they are opened and they come ready to use.

THE CRUX OF GOOD WOUND MANAGEMENT IS TO KEEP EVERYTHING – YOUR HANDS, INSTRUMENT AND SUTURES – AS STERILE AS POSSIBLE. Hands should be washed thoroughly in Hibiscrub, instruments should be boiled for at least seven minutes and the whole bird, except the wound, covered in a clean drape or cloth, preferably a sterile cloth if that can be arranged.

The instruments for a basic suturing kit should be stainless steel and consist of:

one pair of needle holders or Gillies (needle holders that include scissors for trimming sutures)

one pair of dressing scissors

one pair of rat-toothed forceps

one pair of plain serrated forceps

SUTURING

There are many ways of tying sutures, but the best for wildlife work is the simple 'mattress suture', where many doubled individual ties are made along the wound. Then, if one fails, the others will hold – a situation common in skin suturing on birds where there will always be some loss of sutures due to necrosis, or death of tissue.

When a bird comes in to a wildlife treatment centre with a skin wound, there is bound to be damage to some of the blood vessels around the skin edges. Even though they are sutured, some of these edges and skin pieces will go black, dry and eventually fall off. Do not worry too much about this necrosis in birds as by the time it falls off there will be new tissue underneath.

The principle of suturing is to bring the broken skin together, touching edge to edge over the wound. Too much pressure or too tight a

Simple sutures

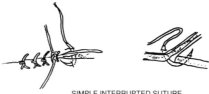

SIMPLE INTERRUPTED SUTURE

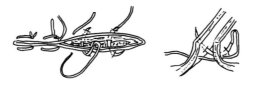

HORIZONTAL MATTRESS SUTURE

knot will also cause necrosis and skin loss. Practising on a ripe banana is a good way to get a feel for the delicate touching of the wound edges. To stop the knot slipping, tie a reef knot with an extra turn in each direction. This will also give a tidy appearance and make the sutures easier to find and remove later. Keep the sutures approximately 0.5cm apart. The ends can be trimmed with scissors or the Gillies.

Muscle tears

These occur most often across the chest and can impair a bird's flying ability. Muscle fibres run in lines and tears may occur across the path of the fibres. They should be sutured together using one of the absorbable sutures like catgut or vicryl. Mattress sutures prevent the additional tearing that often occurs with simple interrupted sutures.

Ruptured crop

A ruptured crop involves both muscle and skin tears. It really is quite a common injury, particularly in pigeons, and usually results in the seed held in the crop spilling out on one or both sides of the neck. This is one of the injuries that needs urgent attention, as the bird cannot take in fluids orally through a ruptured crop and soon becomes even more dehydrated than it might have been before.

The whole area should be plucked and thoroughly cleaned with dilute Savlon or Hibiscrub (see Ch. 2, p. 47). Do not bother to empty the crop completely, but do remove any seeds or other feed that may interfere with the wound.

The muscular wall of the crop should be re-attached to the body wall with absorbable stitches using a mattress suture. If you are worried about blocking the oesophagus (gullet), slide a thermometer or something similar down the bird's throat to show you the route in and out of the crop. The skin can then be sutured normally over the repaired crop wall with nylon or monofilament.

Before inserting the first suture, take your forceps and have a trial run, deciding which edge goes where. Wounds are never symmetrical, never have straight edges and always seem to have too little skin to cover them. However, as soon as you start pulling the edges, the natural way to close the wound will be readily apparent.

As with other skin wounds, the skin sutured over a ruptured crop is very likely to turn black and break down. Do not be tempted to pull it away. Leave it because eventually the skin will regenerate underneath it.

Water birds benefit from a couple of layers of spray-on plastic skin (available in aerosol cans) over any sutured wounds. In general, though, I would not recommend any covering of wounds, not even with powders or ointments and definitely not with bandages or dressings. Healing seems to be much quicker if air is allowed to get to the wound and birds very rarely peck at treated areas.

INFECTED WOUNDS AND ANTIBIOTICS

Although a bird is naturally resistant to infection, cases do occur where some assistance with **antibiotics** is needed. An infected wound smells, whereas birds do not normally smell at all. Wounds that have to be sutured benefit from antibiotic cover, as do all wounds from cat bites. Although antibiotic treatment for catted birds may be a one-off dose, all other antibiotic courses should be completed.

For simple, clean wounds, an **oral antibiotic**, available from a vet, added to the drinking water will hold back any infection. Aureomycin soluble powder (Cyanamid) is ideal but is of little use against an existing infection, which requires a stronger antibiotic. These should be either injected or given by pill or capsule, enabling the dose to be measured precisely, unlike the hit-or-miss method of putting it in the drinking water.

Broad-spectrum antibiotics are usually prescribed by vets, with long-acting amoxycillin being one of the first choices for birds. In mammals, long-acting antibiotics are given every second or third day, but in birds, which have a higher metabolic rate, they must be given every day and in much higher doses per body weight than for mammals. Your vet, who will prescribe the antibiotic, may also be able to demonstrate how to give the injection either subcutaneously or intra-muscularly.

The injection is given with either a 21g (green) needle or a 23g (blue) needle into the right side of the bird's chest. Lay the bird on its back and feel for its breast bone, the keel. To either side there is the muscle mass, which feels like a plump chicken breast, that is so important in judging a bird's condition. On its right side (opposite your left hand) part the feathers to expose the skin. Slide the needle under the skin, keeping it between the skin and the muscle. Pull back on the plunger of the syringe a little to make sure you have not damaged a blood vessel (in which case you will draw up blood), then push the measured dose under the skin. You will be able to see the antibiotic spread and it may leak out as you withdraw the needle. Gently rubbing the injection site will prevent this.

Intramuscular injections are administered to the same site only deeper. If you go too deep you will hit the shield of the keel (breast bone), which prevents you doing any damage to internal organs. It sounds gruesome, but if you are worried, it might be a good idea to practise on a dead bird.

As an alternative to injection, your vet may prescribe **antibiotic capsules** or **syrups**. Syrups can be easily administered by gavaging (see Ch. 1, pp. 38–40) whereas tablets or capsules can be inserted almost into the crop with the aid of a plastic pill giver, available at good pet shops.

At present we are having great success with fighting deep infectious and infected bone injuries by using clindomycin capsules (Antirobe, Upjohn) which are packed in either 25mg, 75mg or 150mg sizes. They are worth asking your vet for, especially for treating birds with compound fractures.

CALCULATIONS FOR DRUG DOSES

When you first start dosing birds your vet will ask the weight of the bird in grams. From that, he or she will be able to work out how much to give and at what frequency. This sounds easy but can be confusing because most drug doses are given as milligrams per kilogram, whereas syringes are marked in millilitres. Luckily, the drug equivalent of milligrams to millilitres is also marked on the product, making a conversion possible.

For instance, 1ml of long-acting amoxycillin contains 150mg of the antiobiotic. The dose rate for birds is 250mg/kg – 250 milligrams per kilogram.

Therefore $\frac{250}{150}$ millilitres per kilogram

becomes 1.66ml/kg

A bird weighing 200g would then receive
$$\frac{1.66 \times 200}{1000} \text{ mls}$$

which becomes $\frac{1.66}{5}$ mls which is 0.33 millilitres

ABSCESSES

Birds very rarely get abscesses, except perhaps for those known as bumblefoot (see Ch. 2, pp. 55–6). Any suspect swelling should be swabbed with surgical spirit and tested by inserting a 21g sterile needle. If there is a trace of pus, antibiotics – long-acting amoxycillin – should keep the infection from spreading. The abscess itself should be allowed to harden and then be incised out by your vet.

SHOT WOUNDS

Many birds are shot but not killed, either by 'sportsmen' or the neighbourhood delinquent with an air gun. Local birds shot with a single air gun pellet usually include pigeons, doves, starlings, gulls, in fact anything that passes within range. Look for matted feathers and a small round hole full of feathers.

Shotgun wounds inflicted by so-called 'sportsmen' involve barrages of lead shot fired from a shotgun, causing any number of wounds. Anything that moves is cannon fodder, including ducks, pigeons, crows, herons, even hawks and dainty waders like snipe and woodcock, together with the intended victims – pheasant, grouse and partridge.

As with other skin wounds, pluck around the wound site (see p. 71), then with a clean pair of fine-pointed forceps feel into the wound and remove the feathers that the projectile will have carried in. It's not always possible to reach the pellet or shot, which can be left *in situ*. More damage can be caused trying to locate it than by leaving it alone. Sometimes, the shot may pass right through the body and be found resting against the skin opposite the wound. These can be simply removed by a vet, who will make a small incision through the skin. Manage any wounds normally with suturing and antibiotics.

Shot wounds to legs or wings do present serious problems in the form of crippling. Even an air gun pellet can and will shatter any bone it meets, adding the further complication of a compound fracture to the wound.

Often parts of the bone are completely shot out, leaving a permanent break which can only result in an unreleasable bird and a possible amputation.

LEG FRACTURES

Most wild bird casualties should be allowed to settle before any treatment, other than first aid, is instigated. One of the exceptions are birds with broken legs which, if left, may try to walk on a fracture, often causing any broken bone to pierce the skin and allow infection to invade the wound, in addition to destroying vital blood vessels and other tissue. A temporary splint may prevent any further damage. And even if your ministrations are too late to save a leg, most birds (with the exceptions of swans, woodpeckers and birds of prey) can exist on just one leg. The loss of both legs, however, is another matter.

Nevertheless, leg fractures heal rapidly and every effort should be made even to save the occasional single leg.

Many cases of 'broken legs' brought into us are either symptoms of nerve or muscle damage, or even head trauma and concussion. A real fracture is easy to identify as the leg below the break site will hang uselessly, often completely out of alignment with the rest of the leg. Above the fracture the leg will function quite normally. Feel the site and you will be able to trace the broken ends of the bones. The bird will feel no discomfort while you are doing this, whereas a mammal suffers intense pain if there is any movement of a fracture site.

If, as often happens, the bone ends are exposed, then clean both them and the inside of the wound thoroughly with dilute Savlon or Hibiscrub (see Ch. 2, p. 47). Then, with sterile forceps, push the exposed bones back under the skin and as nearly in alignment as possible. The inside of the wounds can then be flushed with metronidazole to counter any anaerobic bacteria that thrive in this situation. Suture the skin wound closed and cover with Melolin non-adhesive dressing, ready for splinting.

Some vets may take advantage of exposed bone ends to install a plastic or absorbable intramedullary bone pin to stabilise the fracture completely.

The important thing when dealing with any fracture is to hold it rigid while the healing process produces callus to join the two ends. In birds this can take as little as five days.

Skeleton of a bird's leg

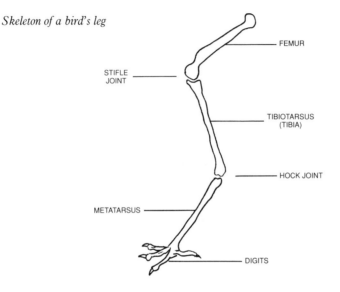

FEMUR

STIFLE JOINT

TIBIOTARSUS (TIBIA)

HOCK JOINT

METATARSUS

DIGITS

SPLINTING LEG FRACTURES

Most leg fractures in wild birds seem to occur in the tibia and fibula, with metatarsal fractures being less common and breaks in the femur fortunately very rare. The femur is covered by the muscle mass of the thigh, which protects it from injury but also makes it impossible to splint. The only sure way of stabilising a fracture of the femur is with orthopaedic surgery and stainless steel pinning or plating.

Fractures of the tibia or metatarsus are treated in exactly the same way – lay the bird on the opposite side from the damaged leg; cover its head with a towel and get somebody else to hold the bird still. You are unlikely to hurt it, so there is no need for any anaesthetics. However, if the bird shows discomfort it may be referred to a vet, who will administer Isoflurane, the only safe anaesthetic for birds.

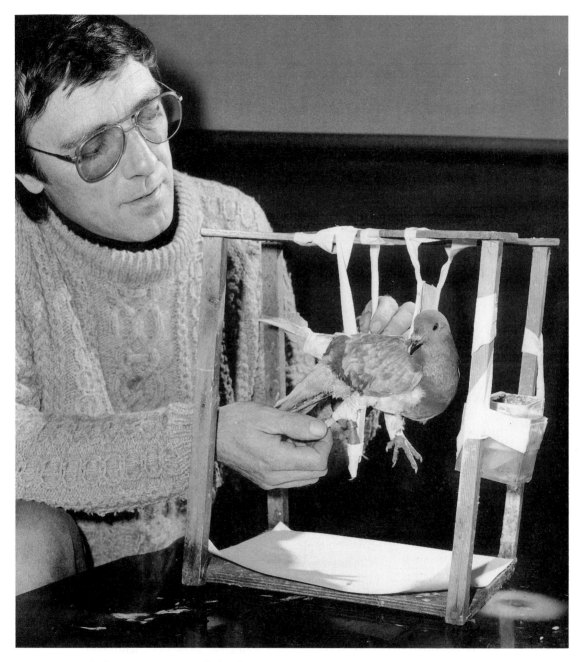

The best way to treat two broken legs

Feel the length of the part of the leg with the fracture and cut a piece of split bamboo or other stick to that length – an ice-lolly stick is ideal. Smooth any ends by covering them with adhesive tape. Cut three or four 15cm lengths of zinc oxide plaster either 1.5 or 3cm wide and keep them handy.

Feel along the fracture site, stretch the leg and feel to where the bone ends meet, with the bones in alignment. Keeping the leg stretched, apply your splint to the part of the leg where the fracture rests against it. Then firmly but not too tightly wrap the leg and the splint with the strips of zinc oxide plaster. Finally, flex the tibiotarsal joint to 90° and apply another strip of zinc oxide diagonally to keep it in place. Check that the foot still feels warm and that your strapping has not compromised the blood supply.

After a week, the splint should be removed to see if the fracture has stabilised. If it hasn't, resplint the leg for another week but do not bother flexing the tibiotarsal joint.

Larger birds, from about 300g upwards, benefit from the pinning of fractured legs, but this is very much the province of specialised avian vets who, at the moment, are few and far between.

Two broken legs

Contrary to a lot of advice given out, birds that have broken both legs can be helped and can recover sufficiently to be released. Quite simply, the bird is suspended in a home-made cradle to keep all its weight off its legs and each leg is treated individually.

Suspend the bird with the aid of crossed strips of zinc oxide plaster, keeping all tapes that pass under the body on the keel (breast bone) and clear of the cloaca (anus). In fact, suspending the bird before you work on the legs makes the whole process of splinting that much easier. Don't forget, though, to put food and water in reach while the bird is suspended.

After a week, check the fractures and if you are not entirely satisfied with their progress, resplint the legs for another week.

When the bird is eventually taken down from the 'sling' it may take a day or two before it manages to walk. Some of the birds we have successfully treated with this system include greenfinches, pigeons, ducks, swans and even herons.

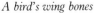
A bird's wing bones

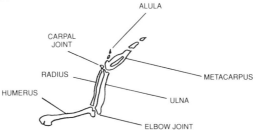

WING FRACTURES

Wing fractures are probably the most harrowing of all wild bird injuries. They must be treated successfully or the bird will never fly again. It does happen that some injuries are probably not going to heal, but in most cases it is always worth trying. Sometimes the healing instinct of a wild bird can produce miracles out of seeming hopelessness.

The wing bones are far more fragile than leg bones and are predominantly hollow, containing a criss-cross of lightweight struts to give strength without adding weight. The humerus, the most difficult bone to treat, also uses its hollow cavity as part of the bird's air-sac system.

Fractures usually occur in just one of the three sections of the wing: the humerus, the radius and ulna and the metacarpus, which I call the 'fingers'.

Fractured humerus

The humerus is the strongest bone in the wing and bears the brunt of the tremendous leverage needed to propel the wings. When a bird breaks its humerus it will quite often continue flapping the stub, tearing muscle and skin in its efforts to fly. Consequently, many humerus fractures are compound. The ideal method of treatment for a fractured humerus is to insert an intramedullary pin, either carbon or plastic – strictly the province of the experienced veterinary surgeon. With a compound fracture this can be carried out as part of the initial treatment, without having to wait for any infection to clear. As birds are so resistant to infection there is a good chance that it will do the job. Even with a simple fracture, your avian vet may decide to pin and wire the humerus, a technique I have seen used many times, especially in tricky birds like sparrowhawks. Even though there is this great resistance to infection, I still insist, in both cases, on a course of antibiotics and have found good results with clindomycin (Antirobe-Upjohn), once again available from a vet.

Because of the positioning of the humerus, it is nigh on impossible to splint a fracture. Without pinning, the only way of stabilising the bone is by strapping the wing to the body with cohesive bandage, which sticks to itself and not to the feathers. When strapping the wing to the body, make sure that any bandage passing under the body is on the bird's keel (breast bone) and clear of the throat and the cloaca (anus). Also, make sure it is not too tight, or it may restrict the breathing. The opposite wing and both legs should be free of strapping and fully manoeuvrable. Then keep the bird confined in a small cage.

After a week check the fracture and exercise the wing joints. If it still has not mended then strap it for another five days and repeat the whole procedure.

Even with a successful repair it may take the bird some time to regain full flying ability and sometimes it may even have to wait for the next moult.

Fractured radius and ulna

These two bones are the bird's equivalent of our forearm. In the event of an accident, they are both usually fractured together. Occasionally only one is broken and that can then support the other, although I do recommend treating it and splinting it as though it was a normal double fracture.

For splint fractures of the radius and ulna, in all but the larger birds, I use the cardboard from cereal packets. Larger birds like herons, ducks and swans will require the more substantial cardboard of a larger box.

Before attempting the splinting, clean up any wounds with dilute Savlon or Hibiscrub (see Ch. 2, p. 47); suture them (see pp. 72–5) if necessary and cover with a Melolin absorbent dressing pad (available from most chemists). The cardboard should be cut to approximately twice the length of the wing, shaped as in the drawing opposite.

The wing should be placed in the rest position, lying next to the body, with the fractured bones aligned to one another. The folded splint is slid

Cardboard wing-splint

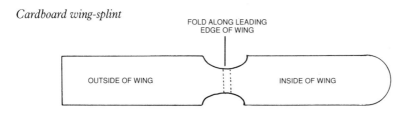

FOLD ALONG LEADING
EDGE OF WING

OUTSIDE OF WING

INSIDE OF WING

on to contain the radius and ulna and the metacarpus – the fold will lie around the carpal joint (wrist). The whole splint is then wrapped in cohesive bandage with a couple of lengths passing around the humerus to support the rest of the wing.

Remove the splint after seven days, by which time the fractures should be stable. If not, resplint for a further five days after stretching and flexing the carpal (wrist) and elbow joints to prevent them becoming stiff. In fact, after the wing has healed, you may have to give these joints a few sessions of physiotherapy to help them regain their mobility.

Fractured metacarpus

Any fractures of these very tips of the wings can be treated in exactly the same way as breaks in the radius and ulna. The only difference is that they will not need resplinting after the first seven days as they will be held securely enough.

Cardboard splint strapped to a broken wing

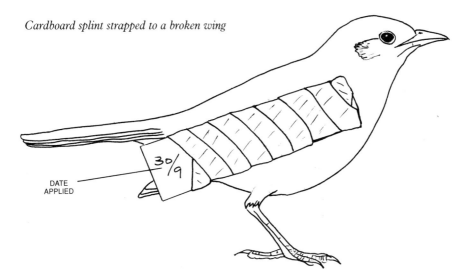

DATE
APPLIED

A *bird's skull*

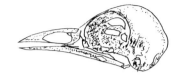

BEAK FRACTURES

Beak fractures are fairly common but are never the same twice. They do not occur in regular positions like those of legs and wings, but can be found at the hinge, just beyond the mouth, halfway along the beak itself or right at the tip, a major problem in woodcocks, which have sensitive mobile tips to their beaks as their main feeding apparatus.

Once again, unless the bird is large, there is nothing the veterinary surgeon can do by way of pinning or plating the lower mandible, where most of the fractures occur.

We have used all manner of ideas on the smaller birds and perhaps a few case histories will explain the level of inventiveness needed to cope with the variety of problems. It's always essential to try, for a bird without the full use of its beak cannot drink; cannot preen; cannot, in most cases, feed; cannot rear young and cannot hope to survive, even in captivity.

Case 19/4/3/88. Blackbird male – fractures each side of mandibles. Beak hanging uselessly.
Remedial treatment: two 21g hypodermic needles were passed through the mandible on each side of each fracture. Nylon suture was fed through the needles which were removed, allowing the sutures to be tied, bringing the two fracture faces together. Left for three weeks. Result: healed.

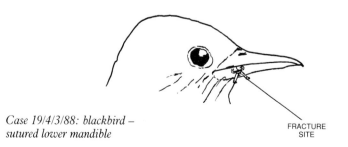

Case 19/4/3/88: blackbird –
sutured lower mandible

FRACTURE
SITE

Case 2/14/9/86. Pheasant male – fracture across lower beak approximately halfway from tip.
Remedial treatment: two wooden splints were placed alongside the beak and were sutured each side of the fracture site. The splint was further supported with Araldite glue. Left for three weeks.
Result: healed.

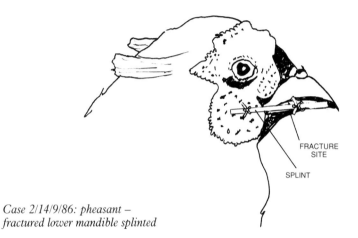

FRACTURE SITE

SPLINT

Case 2/14/9/86: pheasant –
fractured lower mandible splinted

Case 6/27/6/86. Blackbird female – fracture across one side of lower beak approximately halfway from tip.
Remedial treatment: hypodermic needle 21g × 1″ was passed through mandible as support. Removed after one week.
Result: healed.

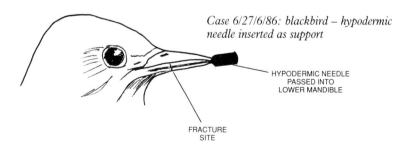

Case 6/27/6/86: blackbird – hypodermic
needle inserted as support

HYPODERMIC NEEDLE
PASSED INTO
LOWER MANDIBLE

FRACTURE
SITE

Case 6/19/10/90. Woodcock – fractures to tips of top and bottom beaks.
Remedial treatment: splinted with plastic splints and tape.

Result: because of necrosis of the top beak, bird was unable to feed and euthanasia was the only course of action.

There is such a variety of beak fractures that each case is different and a test of innovatory skills. Splints and sutures are always useful, so are various sorts of glues and super-glues, but while you are thinking of a solution, sellotape the broken beak shut so that the bird cannot cause it further damage.

Fractures when the mandibles hinge on the skull are impossible to repair directly, but if you can keep the bird's beak taped for three or four days the muscle tension in that area may give enough support for healing to take place. Obviously, during this period efforts have to be made to provide fluids and food, possibly through a gavage tube (see Ch. 1, pp. 38–40) taped in place before the beak is closed. It's difficult but sometimes successful and worth a try to save a bird's life.

DISLOCATIONS

An injury near to a joint on either the wing or the leg that has all the appearance of a fracture may, in fact, be a dislocation. To identify the difference, a dislocation will only involve one bone end, which will feel rounded not sharp, like a fracture site would. True, there could be a fracture close to the joint, but once you get the feel of a dislocation, especially as you try to reduce it, the difference is unmistakable.

The joints most often affected are the stifle joint on the leg or the elbow joint on the wing. Dislocations at the hip and shoulder are best confirmed by X-ray and require complex remedial treatment by an experienced veterinary surgeon.

Dislocated leg joint

A fairly common injury, especially in blackbirds and moorhens, a dislocation of the tibiotarsal joint will present itself as the head of the metatarsus lying by the side of the joint. It is quite a simple process just to stretch the leg and then, with the fingertips, push the bone back into place. The bird will show no signs of discomfort and the leg will function normally again.

As the socket taking the joint is comparatively shallow, the metatarsus may slip out again. Replace it in the joint and wrap it with

Dislocated stifle joint

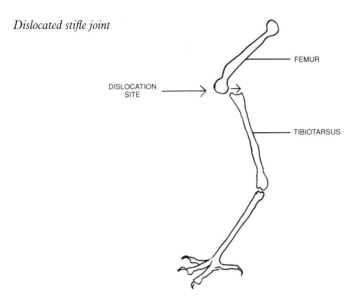

cohesive bandage. This will hold the position but should be removed after a few days in order not to compromise the flexibility of the joint.

Sometimes the dislocated bone breaks through the skin. Clean it and the wound site with dilute Savlon or Hibiscrub (see Ch. 2, p. 47), then reset it. The wound may need a suture and if the joint remains unstable the cohesive bandage should be wound over a Melolin dressing. A short course of antibiotics will help counter any infection.

Dislocated wing joint

The joints of a bird's wing do not have the familiar ball and socket we all associate with a human joint. Instead, there is a very simple meeting of a concave to a convex plane. This makes it very difficult to reset a dislocation and for it to stay in place securely. External support has to be applied until the torn muscles regroup and hold the joint in place.

The joint is easily slid back into place and you should then fully extend the wing to prevent the offending bones from slipping apart again. The whole wing is then encased in a folded sheet of X-ray film, or similarly rigid material like cardboard, which is stapled in place through the feathers with an office stapler. The humerus, radius, and metacarpus are held tight inside the crease of the splint. (Vets can usually supply old X-ray film that has been spoilt or wasted.)

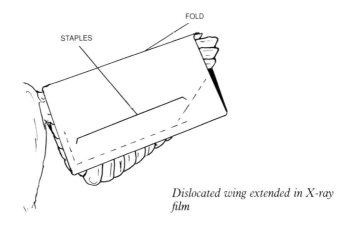

Dislocated wing extended in X-ray film

The splint must be removed after seven days and the joints flexed and unflexed to restore their mobility, remembering that it may take some time and a lot of exercise before the bird can again fly effectively.

AMPUTATIONS

Of course there will be failures, especially where the blood supply has been damaged. Sometimes the bird will manage quite normally but will never be able to be released. If the useless wing or leg proves to be a hindrance, even to a captive bird, then the veterinary surgeon can arrange an amputation.

There is great debate about birds with a leg or wing missing, with claims being made that such a disabled bird would be unhappy, even in captivity. I do not hold with this argument, but appreciate that the future of that bird is really up to its minder. Birds are simple-minded and seem to take any situation in their stride; they do not have the capability of being happy or unhappy. Having said that, I do believe that birds can be depressed and then perhaps the vet should intervene, but even then, the presence of another disabled bird of the same species could make all the difference.

So, before resorting to euthanasia, consider whether the bird might be brighter with company and contact one of the rehabilitation centres around the country, who might just have a similar predicament.

4

Environmental Hazards

including fishing line, oil, tar and other poisons

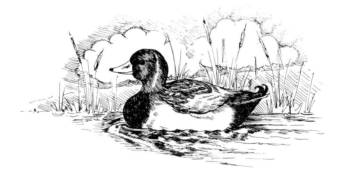

Fishing line

Now that the sale of lead weights for fishing has been prohibited, the sight of lead-poisoned swans slowly dying is almost a horror of the past. But I still see swans and other birds dying from that other blight on the sport of angling – monofilament fishing line, which never rots and once discarded is always lying hidden, waiting to snare the wariest of birds.

Often, with barbarous hooks still attached, monofilament line gets wound around legs, wings, beaks and even tongues, cutting off vital blood supplies, with the resultant necrosis (tissue death) and loss of limbs. Even more horrifying are the deaths of the many swans that have swallowed fishing line only to starve slowly as the hooks, line and weights anchor in and block the bird's oesophagus (gullet).

If the bird is caught in time it is sometimes possible to save its life by removing the hooks and line and starting a course of fluid therapy (see Ch. 1, pp. 35–40) to start to build the bird back to fitness. Sadly, though, even then necrosis of vital organs may make all your effort futile.

Removing hooks and line

The removal of hooks and line from a bird's throat is far less traumatic if one end of the line is still visible at the beak. Clamp that end or tie it to a stick. Do not let the bird swallow it or an X-ray will be needed to trace any hooks and an heroic veterinary surgeon needed to carry out intricate surgery to remove the obstruction. Any line coming from the beak and, if you manage to hold onto it, any hook or blockage, can be removed without the need for surgery. Attach any line showing at the beak onto another length of line or thread using a good knot that won't unravel under pressure. Pass this through a length of plastic tubing that is longer than the bird's neck but narrow enough to pass down its throat. For swans, the most regular victims of fishing line, I use 1cm outside diameter plastic tubing with the ends rounded over a flame.

Lubricate the tubing with KY jelly, liquid paraffin or petroleum jelly and, keeping the line taut through its centre, slide the tube down that line and into the throat and neck of the bird. When it meets resistance it has reached the hook or blockage. Now, very gently, push the hook clear of its anchor point in the oesophageal lining. Gently pull the line into the tubing and, if you have the hook, the whole arrangement of tubing and line should slide free. If it does not slide out easily, the hook may not be clear, so try again to dislodge it.

Never ever pull the line directly out of the throat, as the hook may still snag on its way out. The whole operation, performed by two people with one holding the bird, should go, literally, without a hitch.

The bird has probably been unable to feed and will need fluids and liquid feed to bring it up to strength. Do not offer a starving swan a whole bowl of solid food as it is likely to gorge itself and possibly block its own crop.

OILED BIRDS

We tend to think of oiled birds as those pathetic creatures crawling up the beaches after a tanker has gone down. It does happen, but every day of the year there are birds, often in ones and twos, being polluted on ponds, canals, rivers and lakes. They all need the same tried and tested methods of treatment.

First aid for oiled birds

The first thing to do with any oiled bird is to clear its eyes, nostrils and mouth of oil, using nothing more technical than warmed saline solution (0.9% salt-water) and cotton wool. Similarly, the cloaca (anus) should be cleaned and any matted feathers removed.

Any excess oil can be wiped off the feathers with paper towels, but on no account wrap the bird in anything to stop it preening. We do not want it to preen, but wrapping could cause the major problem of overheating – hyperthermia (see Ch. 2, pp. 59–60). A bird straight from the water with heavy oiling is unlikely to have preened, but a bird on land may have already tried to clean itself and have ingested some of the oil, which is going to cause intestinal problems because of its toxicity.

Before worrying about oil on the feathers, it is crucial to cope with the oil already in the digestive system. Initially, warmed Lectade or International Rehydrating Fluid (see Ch. 1, p. 29) should be gavaged (see Ch. 1, pp. 38–40) into the digestive tract to flush some of the oil through. Calculate the amounts as though you were treating the birds for dehydration (see Ch. 1, pp. 37–8), but as a quick rule of thumb, each bird needs about 5% of its body weight daily – for instance, a 400g crow would need 20ml spread over three doses per day at approximately 6ml per dose.

To follow the first fluids, each bird should be given orally 2–6ml of Kaosal (Loveridge) or one Kaobiotic tablet (Upjohn) to assist protection from any internal oil residues by lining the stomach and intestines.

The bird should then be left upright in a warm container, which could be a cardboard box with an overhead infra-red lamp, for at least half an hour before it is handled again. Birds that are not able to hold themselves or their heads erect should be given an intravenous or subcutaneous injection of dextrose/saline solution (0.18% sodium chloride/4% dextrose) warmed to body temperature. The overall ambient temperature for keeping the birds warm should be between 27–29°C.

Washing

Only birds that are stable, standing erect and looking bright-eyed should be washed. Although it is preferable to wash all birds within 24 hours, those that are weak or depressed should be left until they are strong enough to take the stress of a prolonged handling.

At least two people, but preferably three, should be involved in the washing of each bird; one to hold the bird while the others carry out the washing process. All birds should only ever be washed in a solution of washing-up liquid. (The original choice was Co-op green washing-up liquid, but subsequent experience now suggests that Fairy Liquid produces better results.) Do not try any other product; these work whereas others may produce unforeseen problems, such as leaving oil or detergent residues in the feathers.

Two or three tubs of a 2% solution of the washing-up liquid at 40–45°C (hand hot) should be made ready. The birds should be held in the first tub for 10 seconds and then the washing-up solution worked into its feathers, making sure not to destroy their delicate structure by working in the direction of the feather vanes. The bird's head feathers can be cleaned with a toothbrush dipped in the solution.

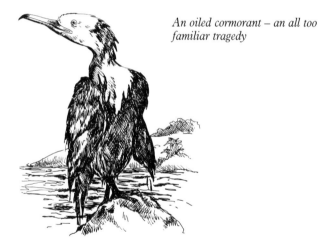

An oiled cormorant – an all too familiar tragedy

When the water is soiled, the bird should be moved on to the second tub and the procedure repeated, and if necessary on to the third tub. The whole washing process should take about 15 minutes, but no longer than 30 minutes.

Rinsing
The bird is then transferred to another tub, this time with clear water, again at 40–45°C. Most of the washing-up liquid and oil floats off and

then the bird is *thoroughly* rinsed under a shower head, once more at a hand-hot temperature. This is the most important part of the washing process, for even the slightest spot of detergent left on the bird could cause it to lose its waterproofing. Waterproofing in a bird is maintained not by any form of oil or substance taken from the preen gland, but by the structure of the feathers themselves being maintained. Consequently, the more that you rinse a bird the drier it will become until eventually, after some time, the water you spray onto the bird will form droplets on the feathers and will run straight off. Only when this condition is reached should the rinsing stop.

Drying

Although the bird will now look dry, it should be allowed to stand and preen under an overhead heat lamp. The bird should be provided with clean water in a shallow container to drink, not to swim in, and various types of food to suit the species (see Ch. 5, p. 104).

Weathering

Over the next few days the waterbirds and gulls should be allowed to swim in a clean pool. At first they will become wet and soon leave the water to preen, but gradually they will restore their feather structure and be able to swim for hours without getting wet or showing any discomfort. They are then, and only then, ready for release in a clean habitat.

Daily treatment

While they are in care, each bird should receive a daily dose of Kaosal or Kaobiotic until their faeces show no trace of oil. Ocean-going birds should, while they are in captivity, receive a daily dose of Nizoral to combat aspergillosis (see Ch. 2, p. 64) and other fungal problems. Also, birds on a white fish diet should receive daily supplements of vitamin B1 to counteract thiamine deficiency brought on by such food.

All in all, the rescue and treatment of oiled birds is a very specialised process, but can be learned by practical experience at an established rescue centre. The best way to become conversant with all the techniques described here could be to become a volunteer at a rescue centre where they have an influx of oiled birds.

TAR AND OTHER CONTAMINANTS

Somehow, birds manage to land in wet road or roof **tar** and are presented to us with their feet matted together. NEVER USE ANY SPIRIT CLEANERS ON BIRDS AS THEY ARE LIKELY TO BURN THE DELICATE SKIN. I have found that Swarfega, available from hardware stores, worked into the tar softens it enough for it to be wiped clear.

Paint can also usually be removed with washing-up liquid or Swarfega. There is only one situation where white spirit seems to be the only answer – there is on the market a non-setting sticky gel that is supposed to stop pigeons or starlings landing on windowsills and ledges. Unfortunately, nobody told the birds, and they regularly land on it, or in it, and are subsequently unable to fly or clean themselves. You will not mistake the gel as neither washing-up liquid nor Swarfega will move it. As I say, white spirit is the only answer for this, but must be thoroughly rinsed off once the bird is clean.

POISONING

Poisons are the elusive enemy of the countryside. Often their presence cannot be easily detected and in most cases we can only surmise that a wildlife casualty has been poisoned. All-too-common cases include herons poisoned with **Dieldrin**, which has run off the fields, and hen harriers, buzzards and eagles deliberately poisoned by gamekeepers and hill farmers. The latter are intentional but highly illegal, as it is a general rule that poison bait, even for poor old foxes, is against the law, and anything suspicious should be reported to the police.

A situation often seen in America but which can happen here too is that of the small bird found suffering chronic seizures after eating poison. Sometimes a minute dose of atropine sulphate from a vet may save a life.

Pheasants and other seed-eating birds may well pick up corn laced with **Warfarin**, put down to kill squirrels. Warfarin has the effect of assisting a victim to bleed to death, often from unseen internal haemorrhage resulting from just a simple knock. Vitamin K injections might help but usually, by the time the victim is found, there is no way to stop the fatal bleeding. Thrush numbers are rapidly declining because they feed on snails which have, in turn, taken in **molluscides, slug pellets** and the like. You cannot diagnose a thrush that has taken in poison but can only support a suspect in the hope that it may recover spontaneously.

There are many **chemicals** innocuously available that are supposed to improve our gardens or our farms. They are all poisons and will kill animals and birds who, thanks to evolution, have a good immunity to natural poisons like yew and ivy.

The one natural poison that regularly rears its head is the bacteria *Clostridium botulinum* – **botulism** being the usual description. This occurs naturally in mud and proliferates when the weather is warm and water levels are low, often affecting ducks, swans and other birds that dabble in the mud. It's also common on rubbish tips, where the household rubbish in black plastic bags is an ideal breeding ground for *botulinus*; rubbish tips are also, unfortunately, a preferred feeding environment for many gulls, and these birds are the usual victims.

The identifying symptoms are a weak bird that is unable to stand yet which has no signs or history of traumatic injury. There is usually a greenish diarrhoea with hardly any smell to it; diarrhoea with a pungent smell points to a **salmonella** infection, which will need antibiotics (see Ch. 3, pp. 76–8). This, though, is unlikely and most cases can be assumed to be botulism.

There are no antidotes to most poisons, but although *C. botulinum* is highly toxic, the majority of birds survive if you institute a broad-spectrum anti-poison treatment followed by good fluid therapy (see Ch. 1, pp. 35–40) and feeding.

A good general broad-spectrum anti-toxin I use is one devised by Andrew Greenwood. His recipe is as follows:

10g activated charcoal
5g kaolin
5g light magnesium oxide
5g tannic acid
all made up with water to 500ml

All these constituents are available from a good chemist and should be gavaged (see Ch. 1, pp. 38–40) into suspect birds at 2–20ml per bird. A swan would have 20ml, whereas a duck could have 10ml and a gull 5ml.

Affected birds would then be offered Lectade to drink, if they are able, or by gavage if they are not. It may take some days for them to recover but with plenty of this fluid 'flushing' they are soon back to normal.

Unfortunately, most poisons have more drastic effects than the lethargy of botulism. All we can do is hope that a bird recovers. However, a little bit of help can be given if a bird is found with its feet and wings clenched in spasm from poisoning. Regular injections of diazepam, given either subcutaneously or intramuscularly, may ease the tension, giving the bird a chance to combat the toxin causing the trauma.

Of course, the best way to combat poisoning is to resist the use of these apparently innocuous chemicals on our gardens and farms.

HAZARDS TO HUMANS

Luckily there are not many **zoonoses** (diseases that can affect man) in birds, especially if you take every precaution with cleanliness, particularly when handling, and do not do some of the silly things I have witnessed – such as kissing birds or keeping them in kitchens where you prepare your own food.

If you develop any flu-like symptoms, or a cough, that needs a visit to your doctor, tell him or her that you have been near wild birds and ask for a chest X-ray just in case.

Infection can be picked up from dusty cages, especially 'bird-fancier's lung'. You can take the extra precaution of wearing a surgical mask when cleaning out bird cages, or else thoroughly dampen the dust and detritus that always collects at the bottom of a cage before cleaning it out. Always wash your hands after cleaning the cage or handling a bird, and do not smoke, drink or eat in the presence of birds.

Ornithosis, the non-parrot form of **psittacosis**, is seen in pigeons and doves and the symptoms are emaciation and obvious sickness, accompanied by conjunctivitis, often only in one eye. It's rare but you may come across it, so it is worth taking precautions if a bird comes in showing these symptoms. Rubber or latex gloves should be worn when handling a suspect bird, as should a disposable face-mask. Keep the bird away from all others and clean the cage thoroughly with parvocide after use.

5

Housing, Feeding and Release

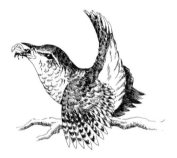

Now that the casualty bird is in care, it needs to be housed in a way that helps its recovery. Incorrect housing can cause all manner of problems.

PERCHES

Firstly, all perching birds should be given the facility to perch or they may well develop foot problems. In particular, I always think that **cuckoos** should have enough perches that they never have to touch the ground. **Woodpeckers** should have logs stood on end or pieces of sacking so they can cling vertically. **Owls** and **hawks** will appreciate an upended log that they can perch on top of. Generally, all perches should be fashioned from natural tree branches; the smooth dowel perches of bird cages tend to be of a uniform width and are totally useless for wild birds, sometimes causing foot problems like bumblefoot and arthritis.

Water birds like gulls, ducks and swans are best off on a soft substrate. Old towels are perfect as these birds do make a mess and towels can be thrown away at least every day. **Wading birds** feel more comfortable on a base of soft soil or leaf litter, gleaned from a local wood. Many of them will only feed if they can probe for mealworms and other insects.

All our other birds are kept on a deep tray of cat litter which keeps dry

99

and absorbs most of the copious droppings for which birds are renowned. Bird sand can be used as an alternative, but I find that it can
cause problems, especially if it gets into a bird's eyes.

CAGING

As a general rule, all cages for wild birds should be totally enclosed,
except for the front, which can be made of normal cage-bird wire or
perspex. Chicken wire is unsuitable as the birds can, and will, cling to it
and damage their feathers. Normal canary cages can be used as a
temporary measure, but must be covered with a cloth or the bird will
panic and try to escape. In the absence of any form of cage, an injured
wild bird could be kept temporarily in a cardboard box with air holes
punched around the bottom. An old towel and a branch or two will give
the bird a chance to stand.

For the new or sick bird there are various types of 'hospital cages'
available, advertised regularly in *Cage and Aviary Birds*, a weekly
newspaper for cage bird enthusiasts. A full range of hospital cages and
accessories is also provided by Sunrise of Rotherham, Yorkshire. These
special cages are thermostatically controlled and are ideal for smaller
birds up to the size of a tawny owl. A good temperature setting for any
sick bird is between 27° and 29°C, but always watch in case the bird
becomes overheated, noticeable by open-mouthed panting or 'throat
wobbling'.

Water birds do not need to swim when first taken in, but should be
offered plenty of Lectade, initially, and then water to drink. This
procedure is particularly important with ducklings, which should not
be allowed to swim until they have grown their mature feathering.
Surprisingly enough, ducklings are not waterproof and if allowed to
swim will soon become waterlogged, chilled and hypothermic (see
Ch. 2, p. 61).

Recovery caging
Once the bird is recovering, standing, feeding and drinking, it should
be removed from its heated cage but still be kept inside for a few days
before going outside. Smaller birds can be kept in **budgerigar breeding
cages**, which are wooden with a wire front. Provide high perches at

each end of the cage to encourage the birds to fly back and forth. Larger birds will obviously need larger cages, but these, unfortunately, cannot be bought ready-made. These birds will probably not be able to fly in their home-made cages but must at least be able to spread their wings. Water birds, not ducklings, can be offered water to swim on; but, believe me, they will make a mess and it is better to resist large water dishes until the birds can be housed outside.

Outside caging

Casualty birds are put outside, both to acclimatise them to weather conditions and to exercise them so that they regain full muscle usage and fitness. Try not to put birds out during wet weather or they may become soaked and cold before they have had a chance to preen their feathers back into order. All birds, except perhaps for the truly aquatic birds, must have the facility to fly, so they must be kept in an aviary with enough space to fly between branches.

Aviaries

All aviaries should be partially covered and should have at least one solid wall where nestboxes or other shelters can be positioned. Welded meshes are available in different sizes suitable for the various species,

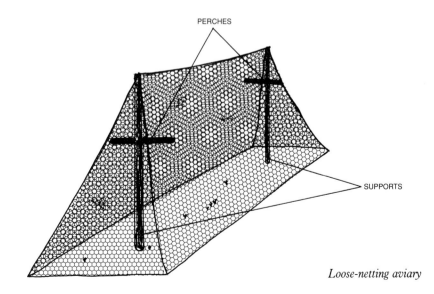

Loose-netting aviary

with the mesh covered in PVC being less likely to damage feathers. Birds of prey, which have the habit of flying at the mesh should, ideally, have an aviary made of vertical dowelling to stop them climbing. However, this form of construction is not entirely practical, so a welded-mesh aviary could be lined with plastic greenhouse shading to lessen any impact with the wire. A new aviary design being tried in America uses a flexible plastic netting fitted at an angle, like a tent. If the bird hooks on to the mesh its tail feathers remain free and will not be damaged.

Nervous birds of prey, like ospreys and some peregrines, hobbies and sparrowhawks, should be housed in a **skylight seclusion aviary** which has solid walls, the only opening being a wire-mesh roof.

Welded mesh comes in different sizes and thicknesses, with the most suitable being:

2.5 × 1.25cm 19g for small birds

2.5 × 2.5cm 19g for little owls, woodpeckers etc.

4.5 × 4.5cm 16g for all larger species

Waterbirds must be allowed to swim and have a pool with a depth ranging from 15cm to at least one metre for diving birds like auks and grebes. Any pool will become soiled, so allow for drainage and cleaning in any pool design. Non-water birds should not be allowed in any pen where there is any form of deep water or I guarantee that they will drown.

Aviary size is very important, and the larger the better. Although it may be difficult to catch a fully fit bird in a large aviary in order to release it, they could be caught at night when they are roosting. A better idea is to have a hatch in a garden bird aviary and release a whole aviary at the same time, holding back those that are not ready for release by catching them before the hatch is opened.

Suggested aviary sizes are:

Small birds to blackbird size: 4m long × 2m high × 2m wide

Pigeons, kestrels, sparrowhawks and owls: 6m long × 3m high × 3m wide

Herons, gulls and large birds of prey: 10m long × 4m high × 3m wide

The addition of baffles, at right angles to the walls, will increase the distance a bird has to fly from one end of the aviary to the other. They will always head for the highest perches, which should be just low enough to give a perched bird a few centimetres' headroom to the roof of the aviary.

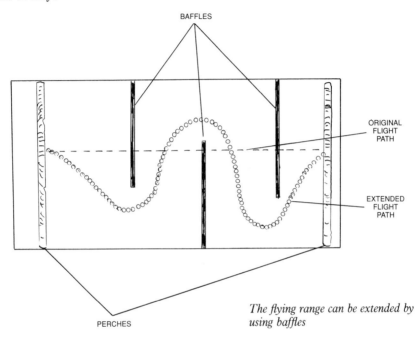

The flying range can be extended by using baffles

FEEDING

For a bird to prosper it really must feed well, so it is essential that its species be identified. I realise this sounds fairly basic, but I know of kestrels that were fed on bread, blackbirds fed on corn and, worst of all, ducks fed on milk. We cannot replicate a wild diet, but by identifying the bird and establishing its normal diet we can at least offer a reasonable alternative. Most of the foods I suggest are always available via advertisements in *Cage and Aviary Birds*. Some substitute foods we use are listed overleaf.

While this book is not intended to address the subject of orphaned birds, a few guidelines on suggested diets may save a lot of birds being killed with bread and milk: all these species are initially reared on St Tiggywinkles glop (see Ch. 2, p. 58) then moved on to adult weaning diets.

Adult diets

Wrens, goldcrests, tits	Greenfly, blackfly, fruit fly culture
Dunnocks, robins, wagtails, waders, hirundines	Natural pinkies (small, clean maggots), mini-mealworms
Blackbirds, thrushes, cuckoos, lapwings, starlings, woodpeckers	White clean maggots, mealworms
Finches, sparrows, buntings, collared doves	Foreign or British Finch mix, wild seeds
Swifts	Force-fed with St Tiggywinkles glop (see Ch. 2, p. 58)
Pigeons, pheasants, swans, partridges, dabbling ducks	Mixed corn
Kingfishers, grebes, fish-eating ducks	Whitebait (with vitamin B1 supplement)
Herons, bitterns	Sprats (with vitamin B1 supplement), *day-old chicks
Auks and other sea birds	Sprats (with vitamin B1 supplement)
Hawks, owls	*Day-old chicks or *mice
Eagles, buzzards	*Day-old chicks, *rats, *rabbits
Crows and gulls	Tinned dog food, *day-old chicks

*Day-old chicks, mice, rats and rabbits are bought in frozen quantities.

All feed should have a multi-vitamin powder added at regular intervals. Maggots, mealworms and corn products can have vitamins mixed as soon as they arrive. All these bird foods can be found advertised in the weekly paper *Cage and Aviary Birds*.

Most other species, except the pigeons and doves, are reared on smaller morsels of the adult diet: e.g. owls are reared on chopped up defrosted frozen mice, ducklings are reared on chick crumbs.

Birds of prey very rarely drink, but all other species should, at all times, have clean water to drink.

Hatchling and fledgling weaning foods	
Blackbirds, thrushes, starlings, cuckoos	Weaned onto white clean maggots or mini-mealworms
Dunnocks, robins, wagtails, hirundines	Weaned onto natural pinkies, mini-mealworms or waxworm larvae
Wrens, goldcrests, tits	Weaned onto greenfly, blackfly, fruit fly or natural pinkies
Finches, sparrows, buntings	Weaned onto small seed mixes
Crows and gulls	Weaned onto tinned dog food or day-old chicks

NON-RELEASABLE BIRDS

The spirit of the Wildlife and Countryside Act allows the rescue of injured wild birds on the assumption they will be released as soon as possible. There are occasions, however, when a bird cannot safely be released due to disability or, unfortunately, its being tame.

These birds can lead a fairly normal life in a suitable aviary and, in fact, may be able to take part in a breeding programme whereby any progeny are released into the wild.

I do not think they should be confined alone to a cage but should have access to other birds of their own species in a community cage. In fact, we have found that some newly arrived casualties will not settle or feed unless another of their own species shows its own familiarity with the surroundings.

RELEASE

Release is the culmination of all the efforts at rehabilitating a bird. If it's done properly the bird will have a great chance of surviving in the harsh world that is its natural habitat. Get it wrong and the bird will not last 24 hours.

We used to have all our birds ringed, with very successful results. However, as rings can cause problems for wild birds – they may cut into the legs – we stopped the practice after three years of positive results.

DIFFERENT SPECIES REQUIRE VARIOUS METHODS OF RELEASE BUT IN GENERAL NEVER RELEASE A BIRD IN AN ALIEN HABITAT.

ALWAYS RELEASE DAY-FLYING BIRDS IN THE EARLY MORNING AND NOCTURNAL BIRDS AS SOON AFTER DUSK AS YOU THINK IS SAFE.

NEVER RELEASE BIRDS DURING ADVERSE WEATHER CONDITIONS AND NEVER DURING VERY COLD, VERY WET, VERY HOT OR VERY DRY CONDITIONS.

ALWAYS RELEASE MIGRANTS WHEN THEY HAVE A CHANCE TO BUILD UP THEIR STRENGTH BEFORE JOINING THEIR CONTEMPORARIES ON THEIR MARATHON FLIGHTS.

Garden birds can generally be released straight into the garden, although it may help a **robin** if you let it go outside another's territory. **Birds of prey** should be 'hacked back' – released in a suitable area but only after having been fed in that area for some time. Once it has gone, food is left by its aviary just in case it wishes to return for a free handout. **Gulls** will fly off from ground level but never let them or herons fly off over water, just in case they crash-land.

Ducks and **swans** can be put straight onto the water but care must be taken that one swan is not put into the territory of another. **Seabirds** like auks and shearwaters should be allowed access to the sea from a beach. Launching them off cliffs could well result in fractures as they plummet to the beach – they are not very good fliers at best.

Think about any release – the bird will invariably fly in the opposite direction from the one you would have chosen. So look out for those hazards: busy roads, stretches of water, territorial contemporaries. And, of course, avoid shooters with their shotguns and air rifles who are likely to halt your attempt at getting a live bird back into the environment – the goal of all wildlife rehabilitators.

PART TWO
Mammals

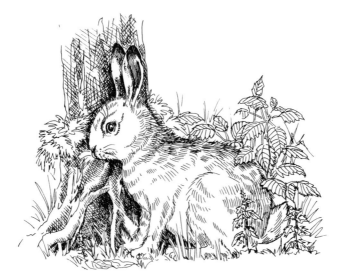

6

Rescue and Containment

Whether to rescue or to leave well alone

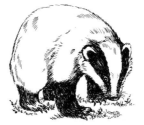

Wild mammals in Britain are, on the whole, shy secretive creatures. We are rarely aware of their presence – unlike a bird's – for when they visit our man-made environment they do so surreptitiously, in the middle of the night. Consequently, most people never see a wild mammal, except for the occasional hedgehog, so they rarely notice if a mammal is injured or debilitated in some way.

The only encounters most people experience are with the flattened corpses on the roads, or with the animal that is finally too sick to hide itself away. Many of the road casualties we are called to have managed by some supreme effort to drag themselves off the tarmac into cover by the time we get to the scene. We then have to undertake an intensive, and sometimes fruitless, search to locate them.

ANY ANIMAL THAT HAS BEEN HIT BY A MOTOR VEHICLE SHOULD, IF AT ALL POSSIBLE, BE TAKEN INTO CARE – ALBEIT ONLY OVERNIGHT – JUST TO ASSESS ITS FITNESS FOR RELEASE.

Many of the faster animals, foxes and deer, are still fully mobile and unapproachable, even on three legs, but if possible these should be caught just to assess the damage to the injured leg, which may or may not need treatment. Either way, the animal will need a longer confinement than overnight.

Assessment is an easy if prickly proposition with a hedgehog (you should wear gloves) but sophisticated or even heroic capture techniques will be needed for squirrels, rabbits and badgers. If you cannot catch the casualty and there is no infection to the damaged leg, then the animal may survive, but any mammal with two legs that are apparently useless *must* be caught. It may be that the animal has a broken back or pelvis, with the consequent bladder disfunction. Even if the casualty survives initially with two broken legs, further damage and infection are sure to follow. I know of a muntjac deer that had two broken front legs but which was still able to run like the wind – until infection brought it down and killed it.

Apart from the friendly hedgehog visiting your garden, any adult mammal that can be approached needs attention of some kind. Situations that spring to mind are rabbits stricken with myxomatosis (with the tell-tale swollen and closed eyes, the rabbit sitting waiting for a predator or death); infected badgers or foxes and dolphins and whales stranded on dry land. They may be approachable for different reasons, but they will all die where they lie unless you intervene.

HEDGEHOGS

There are, of course, exceptions to the 'if it can be approached it is in trouble' rule, notably hibernating hedgehogs, but a hibernating hedgehog will be tightly rolled inside a substantial nest. Hedgehogs do not hibernate in the middle of lawns or uncovered under hedges: these are sick hedgehogs that need rescuing. Similarly, a hedgehog that is out and about during the day has a problem, unless you know that it has recently been disturbed (for instance, by someone digging in a compost heap it was sleeping in). Hedgehogs are strictly nocturnal and only venture out in daylight if they are blind or suffering in some way. Hedgehogs crossing the road at night do not need to be rescued, but if you feel you must help, simply put it onto the verge; do not take it far away – you may be leaving a dependent family behind.

At the end of the year, hedgehogs born in the autumn may not have enough fat reserves to carry them through the winter. It has been established that they need to weigh at least 600g to survive. So if in doubt about an orphaned juvenile hedgehog's ability to survive, weigh it on the kitchen scales and take it in for the winter if it's November or December and the hedgehog does not meet the required weight. It can be fed during the winter and released in April or May, depending on the last frosts; it does not need to hibernate.

Later, during the colder winter months you may come across a hedgehog and wonder why it's not hibernating. If the weather is particularly cold and you are worried about it, take it into a warm room and keep it awake and well fed then release it in spring. It will not have dependent youngsters in the winter and by taking it in you may well discover a problem previously unnoticed.

BATS

You may also come across a bat in the depths of winter. It's probably all right but just in case, offer it a few mealworms then hang it up – its tiny back feet enable it to be hooked to any rough surface – in a frost-free outhouse, where it can make its own mind up about whether or not to hibernate. Injured bats are fairly easy to assess, rather like birds. An obviously damaged wing with broken bones or torn membranes means that it needs treatment, but if no apparent injury is present then try to encourage the bat to fly around an enclosed room. If it can fly, put the bat outside after dark. If it cannot fly it needs treatment and regular hand-feeding with mealworms.

Bats are strictly covered by the legislation of the Wildlife and Countryside Act 1981. This prohibits anybody catching them or disturbing their roost. However, it does allow the handling of bats that are injured or obviously in some difficulty, especially those found clinging to walls away from a normal roost site.

CASUALTIES OF CATS

As with birds, any bat caught by a cat (the most common cause of injury) needs antibiotic therapy (see Ch. 8, pp. 175–6), even if there is no apparent injury. Cats are renowned for their mouse-catching and rightly so. They play a big part in keeping down populations of rats and house mice. However, they also catch field mice, harvest mice, dormice, squirrels, rabbits and even lizards. Any one of these casualties should receive antibiotics before it is released.

Cats themselves are often the victims of snares set indiscriminately in hedgerows. These must go to a vet but badgers, foxes and deer are also regular victims and they, too, obviously need rescuing. They should be held in care for at least a week, even if there is no obvious injury.

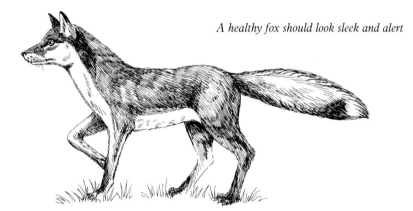

A healthy fox should look sleek and alert

FOXES

Foxes are pretty clever at avoiding most dangerous situations, but they do fall victim to roads and snares. The other problem they seem to suffer from is sarcoptic mange. Some fox visitors to gardens show the symptoms – lack of fur, skin lesions and emaciation. They can and should be treated (see Ch. 7, p. 158). If there is only one regular fox visitor it can be treated without capture by offering food laced with ivermectin from a vet or pharmaceutical merchant; but if there is more than one fox then you cannot simply increase the dose as a blanket quantity to treat the infected one because there is a danger of overdose. Your target fox will, instead, need to be captured and taken into care for treatment.

BADGERS

Badgers are most often the victims of road traffic accidents, but many are seen with horrendous wounds on their rumps and necks. These wounds are probably the result of fights with other badgers and do not seem to cause the victims any concern. There is, however, always the danger of infection or fly strike (see Ch. 7, pp. 152–3) so they will need to be caught and treated. In fact, any animal with wounds is susceptible to these two killers – infection and fly strike – and needs urgent medical attention.

With most mammal species the cause for concern stems from either damage to a leg, skin wounds or lethargy caused by concussion. The other occasions when intervention is necessary are: when an animal is suffering from a disease (myxomatosis in rabbits and mobillivirus in seals); when a casualty is trapped in snares, fences or, in the case of bats, in a front room. It's generally easy to make a decision whether or not to rescue. The only exceptions are apparently orphaned mammals.

ORPHANS

Many mammal species seem to leave their offspring unattended for long periods of the day or night. IN MOST CASES AN APPARENTLY ORPHANED MAMMAL IS BEING CARED FOR AND WILL STAND A BETTER CHANCE OF SURVIVAL IF LEFT ALONE. Typical rescued 'orphans' that were found and which did not need to be rescued include:

Seals
Baby seals are deliberately left on their own and unless very obviously weak, sick or injured should be left alone. If in doubt, watch them from a distance for at least 24 hours.

Hedgehogs
Hedgehog mothers will often not sleep with their young, especially during the day. Once again, watch from a distance for the mother's return. However, if baby hedgehogs – those still with white spines – are found wandering, they will need to be taken into care.

Hares
Leverets are left secreted in tufts of grass. They are born fully furred and should not be picked up.

Deer
Similarly, deer fawns are left alone for long periods and instinctively do not move if you approach. Leave them alone.

Mammal action

When to assist	*When to leave alone*
General	*General*

Animal hit by car
Animal can be approached
  (not hedgehog)
Leg appears damaged
Dragging two legs
Animal has open wounds
Caught by cat
Caught in snare or fence
Any apparent orphan showing
  an injury
Any animal rescued from
  a predator
	All *apparent* orphans except when
	  injured (see species specialities,
	  Ch. 7, pp. 161–2)

Hedgehog	*Hedgehog*
Out during the day Asleep away from the nest Single orphan after surveillance	When in its nest Apparent orphans in the nest
Rabbit	*Seal*
With swollen eyes Single orphan, after surveillance	Single apparent orphan
Fox	*Hare*
With mange Single orphan	Single apparent orphan
Badger	*Deer*
Single orphan, after surveillance Out during the day	Single apparent orphan
Bat	
Cannot fly	
Cetacea	
All stranded whales or dolphins need specialised help	

Foxes, badgers and other mammals

Most of these are raised in family groups. If a youngster is found out and on its own, it may need adopting. But, once again, watch from a distance to see if the parents do recover their straying offspring.

GENERALLY, DO NOT EVEN TOUCH YOUNG MAMMALS, AS THE HUMAN SCENT MAY CAUSE DISTRESS TO THE RETURNING ADULTS.

Lately, **muntjac** or **chinese water deer** have started to visit gardens. They are perfectly all right and should be left alone, as any attempt to catch them will usually result in injury to the animal, and sometimes the human too.

THE CHASE AND CAPTURE

As with the capture of birds (see Ch. 1, pp. 18–19), it's not a good idea to chase a wild mammal, not only because it causes the animal a lot of stress, but also because the chase will probably make any injuries worse. The thing to remember when dealing with mammals is that they are far more intelligent than birds and have a very sophisticated sense of smell that enables them to scent a would-be rescuer, even if you cannot see the animal and it cannot see you. The old hunter technique of being downwind of an animal still holds good, although I doubt if any of us has enough fieldcraft to be able to stalk to within catching distance of an animal that can still run.

An animal that cannot move is easy to approach. You should still keep as low as possible just in case the creature gets a sudden burst of adrenaline, enough to let it get away. This is particularly important with **deer**, which seem to have the ability to come back instantly from the dead and flee on three, or even two legs. Try to predict the animal's reaction even before you approach it. It will have instinctively worked out its escape routes so try to be one step ahead and block these off or use them to your advantage by ambushing the animal as it flees.

Slow-moving animals like **hedgehogs** and **badgers** will not bother with strategy but can still show an amazing turn of speed when they want to. The thing to do is be prepared for their move; you can outrun them and capture them easily if you have the right equipment at the ready.

A **hedgehog** is small and when touched will stop still and start to curl up. If you have stout gloves on you can simply pick it up and carry it into captivity.

However, it's not always that simple. Hedgehogs get tangled in netting, making it impossible to unravel them without anaesthetics. The netting has to be cut away with scissors and the entangled hedgehog taken somewhere that has the facilities to anaesthetise and treat it. Hedgehogs trapped in drains can be rescued with a pair of pliers clamped onto their spines. It's often the only way to get one out of a tight drain and the method only injures their dignity.

In all instances, wearing gloves makes the hedgehog much easier to handle, but in the case of a **badger** they will probably hinder you and will give you no protection from what is the most powerful bite of any British mammal.

ONE POINT TO REMEMBER WITH ALL BRITISH WILD MAMMALS – THE MAJORITY OF THEM WILL BITE GIVEN HALF THE CHANCE. NEVER EVER GIVE THEM THAT CHANCE, TREAT EACH CASUALTY WITH RESPECT AND INTENSE CONCENTRATION.

Quick-release grasper

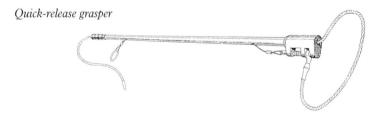

Make sure you have the situation under control and never make a grab for a **badger**, **fox**, **otter** or **seal**, they will bite you quite badly. Smaller biters will have to be handled with *thick* gloves. I use welder's gloves to handle squirrels, *glis glis*, stoats, weasels and water voles. Larger animals will need to be handled with a **grasper** or dog catcher. Quite simply, a grasper is a rope noose coming out from the end of a hollow pole. Slid around the neck of the larger biters, it enables you to bring the animal under control and if used carefully will do no harm. Extra care should be taken with more fragile animals like foxes, cats, martens and mink, but a substantial pressure is needed to hold badgers and otters – they are extremely powerful animals.

Before even attempting to take up any of these animals, make sure that you have by you an **opened crate** or **basket**, so that you can immediately, on capture, put the animal out of reach. Cardboard boxes are not strong enough for any of the biting brigade and badgers, otters and wild cats need **reinforced baskets** (good clean dustbins with secure fitting lids punched with air holes make ideal containers).

British mammal bites

Will bite	*May bite*	*Will not bite* (But don't take it for granted)
Badger	Hedgehog	Deer (but antlers,
Fox	Rabbit (will kick)	feet and tusks could
Seal	Hare (will kick)	be used as weapons)
Otter	Mice	Whale
Squirrel	Vole	Dolphin
Weasel		(but tail flukes can
Stoat		give powerful blows)
Mink		Common dormouse
Pine marten		
Polecat		
Wild cat		
Glis glis		
Rat		

Badgers

Of the large animals, you are most likely to encounter badgers. Their strategy on the roads, or the railway for that matter, seems to be to meet the vehicle head on. Amazingly, many of them survive this, only to lie deceptively comatose until somebody tries to pick them up.

I always approach a badger, with open basket at the ready, with a **thick stick**. I gently prod the head and jaws to see if there is any reaction. If it turns (and they turn like lightning) and snaps at the stick, I retreat for the grasper. On many occasions it shows no reaction, so, holding the head to the ground with the stick, I gather in my right hand a good grip on the scruff of the neck. Unlike dogs, cats and foxes, a badger has very little loose skin over the scruff so it is important to get a really strong grip. Once the scruff is under control it's possible to lift the badger, but before doing so use your other hand to grip the rump, just above the tail. In this way you are not putting any strain on the animal's backbone, which may be damaged. Then simply put your badger in its container, close the lid, but do not release your grip on the scruff until you are sure you can get your hand out without getting bitten.

If you drop the badger on the way to the container do not try to pick it up again immediately. Instead, jump clear and start all over again.

With a livelier badger it is essential to use a grasper. Slide the noose over the badger's head and behind its ears. Make sure that neither of the front legs is caught in it and then pull the noose up as tight as you can. You will not hurt the badger as long as you use a professional grasper not a home-made one, and you will be glad of your grip when you feel how powerful the animal is. When you are happy that it cannot get out of the noose, very, very carefully reach with a free hand for the rump, just above the tail. Pick the badger up, keeping it stretched. It will fight, so as quickly as possible, but under control, put it into the container, close the lid and only then release the grasper. Secure the lid. Badgers will not use their claws to attack.

Otters

Treat an otter in exactly the same way and with the same respect. They are more agile than a badger and can turn to bite the hand that holds the rump, so be particularly careful to keep the animal stretched and the noose as tight as possible.

Foxes

Foxes need similar handling, either by the scruff or with a grasper, but they have a far more fragile neck and it's not necessary to maintain the tight grip used for otters and badgers. In fact, I prefer to handle foxes by their scruffs, getting the grasper off as quickly as possible. Incidentally, foxes will urinate or defecate in fear as you pick them up.

Catching foxes is a bit more involved than capturing badgers and otters, which are, by comparison, almost lumbering. Foxes can run very well on three legs and I remember having to run myself ragged to catch a fox which had only two legs working. Even an apparently dead fox may get up and run, so be prepared for the seemingly impossible. If the casualty is in a garage or outhouse, then make sure there are no exits. In fact, if you want to take an active fox, the best way is to try to persuade it to go into a shed and then jump in yourself and slam the door. Then it is only necessary to slide the grasper over its head – simple in a confined space. In this situation the fox will not normally attack, whereas a badger might.

Outside a confined space it's practically impossible to grasper a fox. It is sometimes feasible to catch it in a large net but our procedure is to set up **'walk-toward' nets**, like high tennis nets, over expected escape routes. These are manned but the people keep their distance in case the fox senses them and veers away. Someone approaches the fox, which flees – hopefully into one of the nets – and becomes entangled. The net is dropped onto it but, as yet, nobody tries to grab the fox as it will bite. Once it is under control, under the net, as with a badger, use a stout

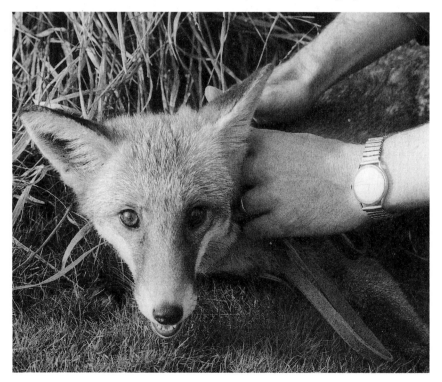

The safest way to handle a fox is by its scruff

stick or a broom to hold the head down while the scruff is gripped so that the fox can be transferred to a basket.

ALWAYS EXPECT THE ANIMAL TO BITE. I will never forget holding a fox by the scruff in a particularly remote wood. I had taken my jacket off in the search for the animal and now I had it; I tried to put my jacket back on (incidentally, I had no basket), which was fine until, with fox in my left hand, I put my right arm through the jacket sleeve and presented fox with a finger, which he promptly bit. I was not concentrating – the golden rule when dealing with any wild animal.

If the fox is too elusive and agile even for walk-toward nets, then the only way to capture it is to use a **fox cage trap**, baited. The fox cage trap is like a large basket with a trapdoor at one end closed by a treadle at the other where the bait, an old chicken or rabbit carcase, is placed.

Deer

Deer are particularly vulnerable to walk-toward nets, with the added advantage that their flight is planless, unlike that of foxes, which think all the time. A fleeing deer will hit the net and all hell will break loose. It's then essential that someone contains the deer before it does itself harm. This is preferably a job for two people, for **roe** and **muntjac-size deer**. Netting is not a procedure I would recommend for red deer because they are too large to handle. Even small deer are strong and can cause injuries with their antlers, tusks and hind legs. With their heads covered with a blanket they can be carried by holding them around the body. Do not try to restrain the hind legs, you can't and are likely to get injured if you are in the way of a flailing hoof. Just let the legs hang well clear of your own legs.

Once the deer is held it should be sedated immediately by a vet with a diazepam or midazolam intramuscular injection before being transferred for transport back to a treatment facility.

If you have to pick up a small deer, then hold it around the middle, do not try to restrict its legs but let them thrash away in mid-air. The hooves are quite sharp and can easily tear clothing and possibly skin. Many of my sweatshirts are stitched up – momentos of encounters with muntjac, which are surprisingly strong for an animal not much bigger than a dog.

All **male deer** will use their heads as weapons. They use their antlers

119

or, in the case of muntjac, their razor-sharp tusks as well, to inflict injuries, if you give them half a chance. Actually, antlers are very good handles for controlling deer heads, although it may take two people to control the head of a fallow buck.

Deer larger than muntjac should always be carried on a stretcher. If necessary, contain the rear end of the animal in a sack before strapping it to the stretcher.

Sometimes it is impossible to catch a deer, even in a net. Then is the time to resort to **tranquilliser darts** fired from a specialised rifle or blowpipe. Before even contemplating such a solution, make absolutely sure that the deer needs rescuing. Some deer with limps, for instance, have been like that for years and manage quite adequately in the wild, and it is doubtful whether you can do anything about a very old injury.

Tranquilliser dart rifles and blowpipes both need Home Office authority and police firearms licences before they can be used. They should also not be used until the licence holder has received proper tuition from someone who is familiar with tranquillising animals and who has then practised repeatedly, albeit into a bale of hay. If possible, get close enough to use a blowpipe loaded with plastic darts. If this isn't possible, make doubly sure that the rifle's air pressure and sighting is correct, so that you do not further injure the deer or fire a dart into the wrong part of the animal. The large muscle mass on the rump is probably the least dangerous site, but any attempt to tranquillise a deer with darts can go wrong so be prepared. More success can be achieved if the shot is taken at a right angle to the animal; a shot from any other angle may ricochet, leaving a dart loaded with drugs lost in the countryside.

The drug of choice, available from vets, for tranquillising deer is medetomidine (Domitor-Norden Labs) coupled with ketamine. The medetomidine can then be reversed with antipamezole (Antisedan-Norden Labs). These are as safe as any anaesthetic or sedation drugs and are not lethal to humans, as is the familiar choice for tranquilliser darts, etorphine (Immobilon – C-vet).

Smaller mammals
Squirrels, **rabbits** and **hares** can be caught with the help of a **large net**, although myxomatois rabbits can usually be approached from behind

and picked up before they realise there is anybody there. A squirrel that cannot be approached will have to be tempted into a cage trap.

On many occasions your casualty animal will have disappeared by the time you get there and no amount of searching the locality gives any trace of it. It is possible to use a well controlled tracker dog to follow a scent, but the dog must never be allowed to get too close to the casualty or the dog may be attacked and injured, especially if the casualty is a badger, otter or muntjac.

TRANSPORTING YOUR CASUALTY

Once contained, most mammals will attempt to escape; but provided the container is strong enough, they should be secure. **Deer** are the most difficult animals to transport, and if possible they should be have their **heads covered** and be **sedated** before any attempt is made to move them. Before it was reorganised and renamed (to English Nature), the Nature Conservancy Council produced a booklet called 'The capture and handling of deer', which suggested a range of different sizes of face mask suitable for various deer species. We have used these to great effect, finding them especially useful for quietening fallow bucks.

Deer should have any leg fractures temporarily splinted (see Ch. 8, p. 179) before they are moved. I carry a range of plastic splints that can simply be bound to a damaged leg with cohesive bandage before the animal is moved. These prevent the deer from doing itself any further damage during the journey. If possible, all deer should be supported upright on their keel (breast bone).

Any **unconscious animal** should be covered with a **towel** or **blanket** and those that are particularly cold and suffering from shock benefit from being wrapped in a space blanket.

ALWAYS CARRY AN ANIMAL IN THE BOOT OF YOUR CAR. It amazes me how many potentially dangerous animals like deer and badgers are carried loose on a passenger seat. I would not like to drive with a deer jumping about behind me inside my car and I distinctly remember having to disentangle a badger from the wiring behind one man's dashboard – it was a terrible mess.

The last rule to remember when thinking of transporting any animal is not even to attempt it on a very hot day unless your car has very, very good ventilation. I know that sometimes rescues have to be carried out in the height of summer, but be aware that it takes very little for an animal to become overheated.

RECORDS

Details of mammal casualties should, like those of birds, be recorded on admittance cards (see Ch. 1, p. 27). Of particular importance is *where* it was picked up, as many mammals have established territories. To release them elsewhere is only putting hurdles in their way by making them try to fight for and establish new homes.

In addition, records can be valuable in aiding statistical research – for instance, we have been taking hedgehogs into St Tiggywinkles that are suffering from a baffling condition: an excess of dental calculus, or build-up of calcium residue, plus its resulting caries and gum disease. This condition could possibly be caused by local environmental conditions. Our record cards tell us where each 'tooth case' was found and so a pattern may emerge, showing areas of pollution or contamination.

INITIAL HOUSING

All mammals are more difficult to handle than birds, so when designing their initial housing remember that they may have to be caught and recaught, especially if they are to receive a course of medicines. Mammals are more receptive to infection than birds, so many casualties will have infected wounds that need courses of antibiotics; they may also be suffering from inflammatory conditions needing corticosteroids, which help to reduce swelling. There is in addition a definite risk of cross-infection amongst casualties, so each should be **quarantined for at least 72 hours**. Many sick rabbits have myxomatosis (see Ch. 7, pp. 159–60), or initially they might just be suffering from severe conjunctivitis. Never take the chance and keep each new rabbit in a **quarantined room** and thoroughly sprinkle each of them with pyrethrum flea powder. Myxomatosis is spread by fleas, and sometimes other biting insects, which must be destroyed. It's also essential to burn the container the rabbit was brought in, to prevent any unpowdered fleas escaping. Myxomatosis will only infect rabbits, although hares may be susceptible. An infected rabbit, or one suspected of being affected, can safely be kept in a room with any species other than other rabbits or hares.

Animals with breathing problems should also be isolated, as respiratory infections can be transmitted through the air – that's how we catch colds and flu.

Other conditions are generally transmitted by contact, notably any of the manges, and if two animals are put together they both need treatment for the same ailment. Leptospirosis is a disease carried by a large proportion of rats and is passed on via the rat's urine. Other species can carry leptospirosis and can infect others in the same cage – the disease can also be transferred to humans. As leptospirosis cases are recommended for euthanasia, the results of a careless introduction can be particularly bad. So, to start with, **keep all casualties separate**.

These considerations apart, I find it daunting enough to have to catch most of the mammals individually for their treatment; the thought of having to catch one while there are others in the same cage conjures up images of escapes and, worst of all, bites from those left behind.

I have had experience of housing most species of British mammal and, if necessary, have built special cages to make handling easier both for me and the animal.

Smaller mammals

The first thing to make sure of is that your animal cannot squeeze through the bars of its cage. You will not have this worry with particularly sick animals and they should initially be kept in a **warm hospital cage** or **cardboard box**. Alternatively, a hot water bottle covered with an old towel is a good heat source, but it does need replenishing as the water cools. Many apparently comatose mammals will start reviving as they warm, and will then try to escape, so any container should be escape-proof from the start.

With lively animals like **squirrels**, **weasels** and **stoats**, always wear gloves and make sure not to allow them even the smallest gap, or they will be out. **Rabbits** and **hedgehogs** are less likely to make a bid for freedom, the latter being easily housed in a hospital cage or deep cardboard box. **Mice** and **voles** are as fast as squirrels and will make their bids for freedom in the blinking of an eye. These are best housed in **plastic fish-tanks** or gallon **ice-cream tubs** with paper towels in the bottom and close-fitting lids with ventilation holes. A small hatch in the centre can be used for changing the food and water.

Bats can be housed in a hospital cage initially – they will climb out of cardboard boxes, but ice-cream tubs will suffice. The best solution is a **home-made box**. In it, the bat can hang on the wall or the roof, has a dark compartment for roosting, coupled by a hatch to a wired compartment where it can feed or drink.

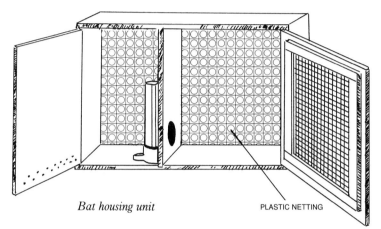

Bat housing unit   PLASTIC NETTING

Do not leave any mealworms or maggots in the housing. Water or Lectade should be provided via a budgerigar 'water fountain' to prevent the bat from drowning in even the shallowest of bowls. All bats will try to bite but it's only with the larger species, the Noctules and Serotines, that it's advisable to wear gloves.

Stoats, **weasels** and **squirrels** can be housed in **budgerigar breeding cages** initially. However, *glis glis* will soon gnaw their way out of any wooden or plastic cage and should be kept in an all-metal cage, preferably one of those designed for ferrets.

Polecats, martens, mink

These three species are strictly carnivorous and are quite dangerous to handle. In fact, we use a large animal grasper to manage mink, a much maligned animal that has now settled into the British countryside without bringing about the devastation of indigenous wildlife that some people had predicted they would. These species should be held in **secure cages**, preferably those with a central hatch in the top rather than a front opening. They do not gnaw so can be kept, albeit temporarily, in specially made wooden boxes – something on the lines of a tea chest with a wire front.

Specialised cages and baskets have been designed for **feral cats**. These have a 'crush' facility that enables you to pull the animal to the sides so that if an injection needs to be given there is no need to wrestle with the animal directly. Injections could be administered to sedate or anaesthetise, either of which is necessary for examining any of the larger mustelids. Or it may be that you need to give a routine antibiotic or worming injection.

Badgers and otters

Badgers and otters are particularly large and powerful mustelids. Their caging must be of at least 10g wire mesh and they do need a crush facility if you are to have any chance of successfully handling or treating them. Unfortunately, they are too powerful for a cat crush-cage. Recognising our need for a stronger version, MDC of Luton now manufacture, to our dimensions, a crush-cage strong enough to hold badgers. After initial examination and treatment of these larger mustelids, they must be transferred to more **spacious cages**. We use stainless steel recovery pens, but in the early days of the wildlife hospital we used any cage that seemed strong enough to hold them, even resorting to solid wooden boxes, tea chests and clean dustbins, when I rescued nine badgers over one weekend and ran out of conventional containers. Handling in a more spacious situation does require the use of a grasper, or a stick and scruffing if the animal is particularly weak.

Injections in this situation are by stealth, the animal confined by holding its head with a stick or broom. But usually, after any initial treatment, we dose all our badgers, and foxes for that matter, by secreting antibiotic pills in their food.

Deer

You cannot secrete pills in the food of deer, for they should never be given antibiotics by mouth as these will destroy the animal's natural gut flora. Antibiotics should always be injected. This is not too difficult when you have a sick muntjac lying down in a box, or other large cage. But when it is a standing deer, there will inevitably be a struggle, possibly causing injury both to the handler and to the deer.

The four deer species that are regularly taken into care are **fallow**, **roe**, **muntjac** and **Chinese water deer**. At the moment, most red deer are confined to private parks and remote high ground, effectively keeping them away from the three hazards the others are likely to encounter – roads, fences and dogs.

Deer are quite highly strung and if possible should be kept sedated with diazepam or midazolam or – a recent suggestion for long-term sedation – pipothiazine palmitate (Piportil Depot, M&B), available from a chemist on the prescription of a vet. This, of course, is not always possible, but it is still important to prevent the deer damaging themselves in their frenzy. If they are given any space at all they will inflict terrible injuries on themselves.

Our remedy for the small species, **muntjac** and **Chinese water deer**, is to keep them closely confined in **wooden containers with chain-link tops**. Access is through the hinged top, enabling a handler to control the deer's head first. The box should be barely a centimetre higher than the deer's upright head or antlers – the suggested height is 65cm. Giving it any more height results in the animal springing upwards, damaging its head and legs. The other dimensions can vary from 1.5m to 2m in length by 66cm front to back. A wooden base is essential to enable the deer to gain a decent foothold.

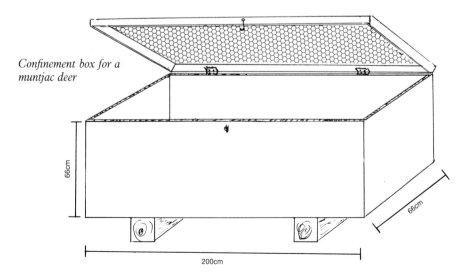

Confinement box for a muntjac deer

66cm

66cm

200cm

It's not always practical to keep the larger deer, such as full-grown fallow bucks, since the size necessary would be that of a small shed. Therein lies the solution – a **wooden shed**, illuminated by a red light, which does seem to soothe deer. Before they have settled or been sedated, the deer's eyes are covered with a mask and its antlers wrapped in foam rubber, just in case it manages to catch someone unawares.

Handling deer is always a problem, but one man can just about hold a muntjac buck, I would suggest two for a roe deer and at least three for a fallow buck, with at least one on each antler. This all sounds a bit traumatic so I would strongly suggest that anybody wishing to handle the larger deer should obtain Home Office authority, coupled with a police firearms licence so that they can use a blowpipe with a tranquilliser dart (see p. 120).

Incidentally, deer should always be supported upright on their keel (breast bone) if they are unable to support themselves. If you have to lay them down, put them on their right side only, to allow their complicated digestive system to function properly, but get them back on their keel as soon as possible.

Foxes

Compared with deer, foxes are very easy to contain and can be kept in **strong metal or wooden cages**. A crush facility would be an advantage for early treatments but after that a cage made out of two tea chests joined with wire mesh across one end would suffice as a temporary holding facility. Foxes can jump to tremendous heights and are particularly clever at escaping, so exercise extreme caution when opening any fox cage.

INITIAL FIRST AID FOR MAMMALS

In general any injured wild mammal should be kept warm, either by covering the larger species with blankets or placing the smaller ones on covered hot-water bottles in boxes. Some initial measures should be taken to settle the animal and keep it alive before assessing its problems, which can be dealt with either by using the first-aid measures listed over the next few pages or for the treatment for the more specific conditions (see Ch. 8) by referring the casualty to a vet.

Mammals are less easily stressed than birds except, perhaps, in the cases of deer and hares – animals which are totally scatty. Their wounds and infections are not necessarily freshly inflicted as, unlike birds which are instantly grounded by wing injuries, many mammals can carry on for many weeks with a damaged limb until finally any infection brings them down. Be prepared for evil-smelling wounds and abscesses, which are common in mammals but rare in birds.

Animals such as **deer** and **hedgehogs** may need anaesthetising before any wounds can be cleaned, but your vet will have to evaluate the danger of an anaesthetic as opposed to leaving the animal for 24 or 48 hours so it can be rehydrated and stabilised.

Foxes and **badgers** can be muzzled with a 5cm cotton bandage – a vet will show you how. When using this system, the animal's front legs must be held under control or else it may pull the muzzle off. It's also a good idea to put two muzzles around a badger's short snout, one over the other, for strength.

Some checking procedures should be carried out as soon as the animal is taken into care. These are:

1 Can the animal breathe?
Extend the neck. Clear the nostrils and pull the tongue forward.

2 Is there bleeding?
Any small haemorrhage can be stemmed with a pad of sterile gauze, a caustic pencil or dilute potassium permanganate (available from chemists). Copious bleeding should be stemmed with a pressure pad or, if bleeding is from a leg, with a tourniquet which should be released every fifteen minutes. Urgent veterinary intervention is needed for any animal with serious blood loss. Of course, there is bound to be some kind of wound but be careful about cleaning it or you may start it bleeding again. If you are happy that any bleeding has finally ceased, then refer to Chapter 8 on ways of cleaning and closing the many types of wound likely to be encountered.

3 Is the animal dead or unconscious?
Give it the benefit of the doubt or listen for any heartbeat with a stethoscope. A stethoscope is always handy and can be picked up very

cheaply. If you don't have one then use your fingers to feel for a pulse, especially in the soft tissue under the forelegs. A vet can prescribe corticosteroids to lessen the impact of a concussive injury but could withhold these if there is fear of any infection being present.

4 Is the animal actually breathing?
Regular pressure on the lungs may encourage an animal to start breathing again. **Do not give the 'kiss of life'** because of the risk of zoonoses, diseases which can be passed to humans. An endotracheal tube can be placed and coupled to an oxygen source through a re-breathing bag by the vet. Regular dilating of the rebreathing bag may stimulate breathing again but do remember that it is the level of carbon dioxide in the body's system that stimulates breathing. If the body is flooded with pure oxygen, the stimulus is not there and the animal will not breathe on its own. Dopram drops, available from a vet, under the tongue may help an animal start breathing again if applied immediately it stops breathing.

5 Are the eyes damaged or not closing?
Damaged eyes should be coated initially with a bland chloramphenicol ointment, available from a vet, and referred without delay to a vet experienced in ophthalmology.

An unconscious animal may not be able to close its eyes, resulting in unnecessary damage by drying out. Regular applications of hypromellose drops, from the vet, or a daily coating of Lacri-Lube ointment, available at chemists, applied inside the lower lid, should protect them until the animal recovers its full mobility.

6 Are there any leg fractures?
Unlike fractures in birds, those in mammals are very painful and no manipulation should be attempted without the use of anaesthetics. Compound fractures should be cleaned and treated immediately, whereas simple fractures can wait until the animal is stabilised and X-rays are available. A temporary plastic splint held in place with cohesive bandage will give some stability until the vet can attend. BONE INJURIES IN MAMMALS SHOULD BE REFERRED TO AN EXPERIENCED VET AS SOON AS POSSIBLE.

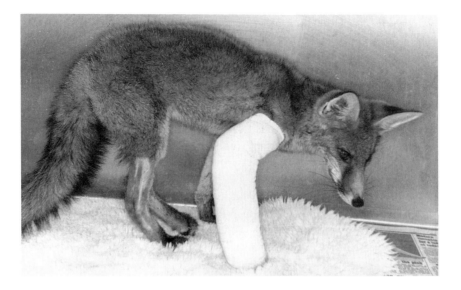

Fractures cause mammals great pain and should be referred to a vet as quickly as possible

7 Are the back legs working?

If not, then suspect a broken back or pelvis. Keep the animal as steady as possible and use a stretcher. Sedate it to stop any unnecessary movement and get it to X-ray as soon as possible.

Often, **bladder malfunction** is a result of this kind of injury. Paralysed bladders in small mammals should be **emptied twice daily** by gentle pressure. Feel in the lower abdomen for a hard balloon, which is probably a full bladder. Squeeze it very, very gently and urine should come from the penis or vulva. Any vet is trained in this procedure and, I am sure, will give instruction on this very delicate, life-saving procedure. An unemptied bladder can, within 24 hours, lead to kidney failure and a dead animal.

Larger mammals may benefit from a urinary catheter, once again fitted by the vet.

8 Fly strike

During the warmer months any mammal with an open wound is susceptible to **attack by blowflies**, which lay their eggs, which hatch into **maggots**. *All* of these must be removed immediately and the wounds flushed with dilute Savlon (barely colouring the water) or Hibiscrub. If it is not advisable to work closely on a wound for a length of time because the animal is too dangerous, then the wound can be packed with Battle Fly and Maggot Paste, available from agricultural dealers.

Check maggot wounds two or three times a day for three days just in case even one maggot has been missed. Treatment with ivermectin, available from pharmaceutical merchants, will control any strays.

Other ectoparasites, such as fleas, ticks and lice, should be left. They are not going to kill the animal, whereas an insecticide might.

9 Are there any strange lumps?

These could well be **abscesses**, reservoirs of infection that are extremely painful. Clip the hair, or spines, over the lump. Swab it clean with surgical spirit and then pierce it with a sterile 21g hypodermic needle. If there is pus present it will show as white at the puncture site. If this is the case, the hole should be enlarged and all the muck squeezed out. Flushing the empty abscess with dilute hydrogen peroxide, available from chemists, will dislodge any material not cleared initially, then a final flushing with a weak Savlon solution or Hibiscrub will remove any particles.

The abscess may well form again and will need cleaning every day until the skin over it recedes or else sloughs off. Abscesses should never be covered and must be kept open so that they can drain.

10 Deer

Deer are notorious for dying at the first opportunity. They suffer from a condition called **post-capture myopathy** for anything up to two weeks after confinement. I have found it successful to give every new deer casualty a massive injection of the corticosteroid, dexamethasone, from a vet. Doses for a muntjac are 3ml, with larger deer, such as a large fallow buck, having up to 15ml. Midazolam or diazepam, also from a vet, will also help calm the animal.

11 General first aid

Any mammal that arrives with an infection of any sort should start a course of injected antibiotics as soon as possible. Amoxycillin is a good broad-spectrum antibiotic, but rabbits should have a preparation not based on penicillin as they exhibit adverse reactions to this antibiotic. Borgal (Hoechst) is appropriate.

UNLESS YOU ARE VERY EXPERIENCED, I WOULD RECOMMEND THAT EVERY
MAMMAL CASUALTY IS SEEN BY A VET AS SOON AS POSSIBLE.

FLUID THERAPY

This is based on the same guidelines advocated for the loss of body fluids
in birds (see Ch. 1, pp. 35–40). Mammals seem to be more susceptible
to dehydration, however, and every casualty will need support of some
kind. Thankfully, many mammals, on arrival, show a willingness to
drink Lectade. However, it is always worthwhile considering the extra
administration of fluids through the various routes available in mammals, once you have estimated the degree of dehydration.

Estimate of dehydration in mammals	
Clinical signs	*Estimated % of dehydration*
No obvious signs of dehydration but a history of fluid loss and assume all casualties have some deficit.	4%
The skin appears tight. Mouth is dry, eyes starting to dry.	5%
Mucous membranes in mouth are dry and red. The skin appears even tighter. Eyes beginning to sink. Urine concentrated and reduced in volume.	6%
Pulse very weak. Eyes, sunken, pinched skin forms tents, hardly any urine, mucous membranes pale, capillary return slow. A very sick animal.	8%
Animal very cold. Eyes shrunken. Animal almost comatose. Skin remains tented. Mucous membranes pale. Life threatening.	10%

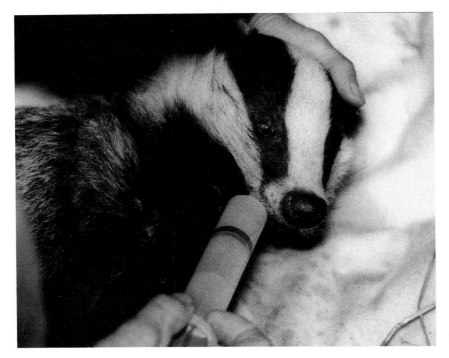

Every casualty will need some form of fluid replacement

How much should be given? There is only one guaranteed way of accurately assessing fluid losses – the calculation of packed cell volume from a blood sample spun in a centrifuge machine. This, of course, is probably the domain of the vet who may have the requisite equipment.

It is possible to estimate the amount of fluid lost through diarrhoea or vomiting but, in my opinion, it is more reliable to use the following guidelines shown opposite.

When an animal's skin is pulled up in a pinch it will normally spring back flat. As dehydration increases, the return becomes gradually slower until, in severe dehydration, it remains tented.

The mucous membranes, which are in fact the gums, are fed with blood through capillaries. These are the first to be shut down in shock and although they would normally appear deep pink, they become paler as dehydration increases. Pressing the mucous membranes with a finger blocks the capillaries which should refill the instant your finger is removed. This response also becomes slower as dehydration takes over. These are good tests to establish dehydration which, with the other typical signs, allow a calculation of how much fluid needs to be replaced.

For instance, a fox is found with chronic mange. It obviously has not eaten or drunk anything for some time. Its eyes are sunken and its skin is 'drum tight' around its body. It makes no response as you pick it up. This animal could be dehydrated by 10% or more. It is close to death and needs fluid replacement urgently.

Weigh the fox – 4.5kg

Therefore fluid deficit is 4500gm × 0.10 = 450ml

Added to this, it also needs maintenance fluids at 50ml/kg per day
= 225ml

This fox therefore needs 675ml of fluid.

It would be impossible and inadvisable to try to get all this fluid in during the first day, so the deficit of 450ml can be spread over two days, in addition to the maintenance of 225ml on each of these days. These calculations are very simple, but the vet may want to include plasma replacements and other sophistications and in fact should always be consulted for animals in this chronic condition.

Types of fluids

There are two basic types of fluid available as replacements, for simple administration to wild mammal casualties. As in birds (see Ch. 1, p. 36), fluid that has been lost over a period of time can be replaced with 4% dextrose and 0.18% sodium chloride available from most veterinary practices, whereas rapid fluid losses through bleeding, diarrhoea and vomiting can be countered with Hartmann's Solution, also available from most vets. An addition of 10% Dephalyte (Duphar) to fluids will help replace lost amino acids and other vital minerals and vitamins.

If the animal shows a willingness to drink then any therapy would be assisted by the rehydrating fluid Lectade (Beechams), available from veterinary centres. International Rehydrating Fluid (see Ch. 1, p. 29) is also suitable if Lectade is not to hand.

MILK, BRANDY, WHISKY AND EVEN WATER, GIVEN TO A DEHYDRATED ANIMAL MAY CAUSE SEVERE COMPLICATIONS THAT CAN KILL THE PATIENT.

All fluids should be warmed to about 37°C before administration by whatever means.

How to give fluids

Unlike in birds, it is inadvisable to try to force-feed mammals with oral fluids. The three routes of administration in mammals depend a lot on the size of the animal. The preferred route is intravenously, but it is really not practical in any animal smaller than a fox, owing to the small size of their veins.

Intravenous fluids are the most rapidly absorbed, followed by fluids given **intra-peritoneally**, that is, directly into the abdomen. However, unless this method is carried out meticulously, and only then in a comatose animal, there is a danger of damaging abdominal organs or causing peritonitis.

Subcutaneous fluids. Although not the most effective, these are certainly the easiest to administer. After calculating how much fluid is needed, this amount is drawn into a syringe and warmed to body temperature. The skin on the back or flanks is pinched up between three fingers and the needle slid under the skin parallel to the surface. Aspirate, (that is, pull back the plunger to make sure the needle has not damaged a blood vessel – if you have you will draw up blood) then expel some of the fluids under the skin. Do not put all the fluid dose into one site as it may cause necrosis, or dying off, of the overlying skin; rather, use several sites across the back and flanks.

Subcutaneous fluids can be given to hedgehogs by sliding the needle under the skin on the bare patches between the spines. Most vets would be happy to show how to administer subcutaneous fluids and will also supply the necessary fluids, needles and syringes.

Intraperitoneal fluids are particularly useful for a small animal that is in shock, cold and near to death. Administration should not be attempted without instruction but, basically, a 22g intravenous catheter is entered into the abdominal cavity making sure not to enter any of the abdominal organs. Warmed fluids can then be given through the catheter, which can be left *in situ* for further administrations until the animal has recovered enough to drink fluids from a bowl.

Intravenous drip. This is by far the most effective route of administration of fluids and a dramatic lifesaver. The veins used are usually the cephalic veins over the front legs; the jugular (in the neck) or the femoral (over the back legs) veins are larger but more awkward to utilise. Placing an intravenous drip is a two-person exercise and should not be attempted unless under instruction from the vet. It will save the lives of otters, seals, foxes, deer, badgers and other large mammals, so I would recommend adding fluid administration kits to any first aid equipment.

Fluid administration kits, for use by the vet, would include:

Giving sets
20g × 1¼″ 'over the needle' catheters
22g × 1″ 'over the needle' catheters
20g × 2″ 'over the needle' catheters
1″ adhesive plaster
2″ cotton bandage
1″ cohesive bandage
Curved scissors or electric clipper
Cotton wool
Surgical spirit
Litre bags of 4% dextrose 0.18% sodium chloride
Litre bags of Hartmann's Solution
Litre bottles of Haemaccel plasma volume expander
2 litre jug for hot water
Selection of sterile scalpel blades

The rate of drip of intravenous infusion is critical and can cause excessive fluid in the lungs if allowed to run too quickly. The vet will advise on drip rates, i.e. how many drips per minute, and this must be monitored closely or the animal may drown. St Tiggywinkles produces a wall chart giving the flow rate used in different sizes of animal.

The one drawback of intravenous fluid administration is that foxes, for instance, will regularly bite through their giving set. As the set runs directly into a major vein there is a possibility that the fox could subsequently bleed to death. Plastic Elizabethan collars may work on dogs and cats to prevent this kind of accident, but foxes and badgers are out of them as soon as their condition improves. Close monitoring and regular checks of the animal are really the only precautions that can be taken to prevent fatal accidents.

7

Assessment and Treatment of Injuries

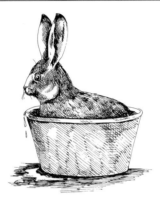

With the possible exception of a hedgehog, any mammal that allows itself to be caught is in trouble. And worse still, if it has not been trapped either intentionally, with snares, accidentally with wires, hit by a car or caught by a cat, then it's safe to assume that its vulnerability is due to advanced infection of some kind.

Unlike most birds, mammals show a strong will to survive and will continue to live even through the most horrendous injuries. However, infection or starvation will eventually bring them down and only our intervention gives them any chance of recovery.

You can tell if a bird is going to recover or die, often within 24 hours, but some mammals on intensive treatment may not show improvement for some weeks. I have known badgers to show no interest in food for three weeks and then start eating, and a fallow buck with concussion that acted blind for 15 days until, in an instant, he was up and seeing and raring to go.

Luckily, the veterinary profession receives intensive training on mammal ailments and conditions, so their first principles can often be applied and their drugs used to assist any casualty. Unlike domestic animals, however, wild casualties have no history of affliction, their injuries or infections are mostly long-standing and you cannot succour a wild animal by cuddling it or patting it on the head. It is on its own, frightened and aggressive; it does not know that you are trying to help.

In spite of this, the animal still has to be handled, albeit under sedation or anaesthetic, to try to identify if there are problems other than the obvious broken leg or damaged mouth.

Mammal skeleton

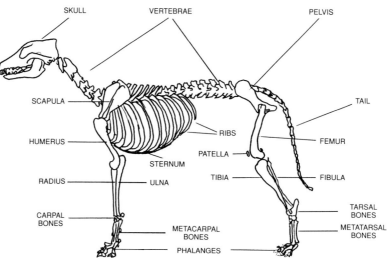

INITIAL ASSESSMENT

Take a look at the animal before handling it.

Is it able to stand? Make it move, if it can, and take a note if it does not use one of its legs. Does it try to use the leg or does it just hang uselessly?
Are the animal's eyes bright and its nose clean?
What is the condition of the fur?
Are there any traces of blood?
Has it urinated or defecated?
Does it try to bite?

These are all important pointers to possible injuries or conditions. Keep a check list for each animal and before you even pick it up, have a space for 'possible diagnosis' – sometimes the first opinion is the most accurate.

Of course, this 'possible diagnosis' needs to be confirmed by closer examination and the animal may have more than one thing wrong with it. We have just released a fully recovered fox that obviously had mange and a damaged tail but a closer examination also revealed old bite wounds on its hip and several teeth needing dental treatment, both of which took a lot longer to rectify than the obvious problems.

Many mammals will actually need you to go out and rescue them. But whether the animal is picked up on a rescue or arrives in a cardboard box, it's still very helpful to pose the questions as to how it came to need rescuing; the following questions and their answers may well give a guide to an injury, like concussion, that is very hard to identify, even on close examination (see table overleaf).

HANDLING UNCO-OPERATIVE MAMMALS

Before any examination or treatment of any but the weakest mammals, it may be necessary to restrain the animal in some way both for its own good and for the handler's safety. There is always brute force but this only adds to the stress felt by both the animal and the handler.

Some animals are receptive to examination and make no attempt to struggle or bite except, perhaps, if there is a painful condition. Others will need restraining even before the vet administers a sedative or anaesthetic. Most biting animals can be muzzled with 5cm cotton bandage or preferably held in a crush-cage (see Ch. 6, p. 125) where the vet can inject a suitable drug to quieten the animal.

For most mammals, the vet can inject a cocktail of medetomidine and ketamine to bring about temporary anaesthesia, which can be reversed with atipamezole. The anaesthesia can be prolonged with Isoflurane inhalation anaesthetic. **Hedgehogs** and other small mammals can be anaesthetised directly through an Isoflurane system. **Deer** can be anaesthetised with medetomidine and ketamine but may be manageable on injections of diazepam although this has no analgesic qualities. Particularly irascible deer can be sedated over a lond period on one injection of pipothiazine palmitate (Piportil Depot – M&B), which could quieten the deer for two to three weeks. A note though – it may take 72 hours to have any effect.

These anaesthetics are strictly the province of the veterinary surgeon,

Questions for the mammal rescuer	Action
Was the animal found on or near a road?	Look for concussion, fractures, head and jaw damage and abdominal injuries.
Was the animal caught by a dog or cat?	Treat with antibiotics. Dog injuries could include skin tears and fractures. Cats inflict skin tears on immature animals like baby rabbits and squirrels.
Was the animal caught in netting, wire or a snare?	Animal will be dehydrated. Remove all traces of ligatures and check for infected skin wounds (see Ch. 8, pp. 172–3). Observe for at least seven days for skin eruptions.
Is there a suspicion of gunshot wounds?	Check for blood on the fur. X-ray.
Is there any history of crop spraying, insecticide or slug pellet use in the vicinity?	Could point to some kind of poison (see pp. 163–4). Look for hypersensitivity, muscle spasms or drooling at the mouth. The latter could also indicate a mouth injury.
Did the animal come from a managed woodland?	Pale mucous membranes (gums) could indicate Warfarin poisoning.
If a squirrel, was it found under a tree?	Possibly a fall, look for fractures, concussion and usually a bloody nose (see Ch. 8, pp. 178–83).
Has the hunt been around recently?	Could be the cause of exhaustion myopathy in deer, foxes or hares.
Was the animal uncovered in a compost heap or other pile?	Look for punctured skin wounds or burns (see p. 147), if there has been a fire.
Has the animal been sprayed for fleas?	Completely unnecessary, this can cause complications to any existing condition.

Assessment of the animal itself

Is the animal able to stand without assistance?	If not look for leg, pelvis or back injuries, concussion, dehydration, poisoning or just general weakness.
Is the animal holding one leg up or is it hanging uncontrolled?	An uncontrolled leg may be fractured. If not look for muscle or nerve damage, abscesses, over-length claws (remember badgers and hedgehogs have very long claws). Foot damage, a thorn or grass spike may make the foot sore.
Are the eyes bright, round and not shrunken?	If not, assume dehydration.
Does the animal respond to your approach?	If not, suspect either infection, dehydration or concussion.
Is the animal shivering?	Could obviously mean hypothermia but, I believe, badgers shiver in rage.
Does the animal smell differently from its normal species scent or does it smell 'bad'?	Infected wounds and mouths will give off a suppurating smell.
Is the animal defecating and urinating? Does it have diarrhoea?	The mucky end but essential in establishing dehydration or a damaged bladder. Could there be a stomach upset?

however practically every hedgehog casualty needs unrolling as it is normally impossible to hold one open to treat leg or body wounds, so if there are a great number the vet may advise on a suitable system to save dozens of visits to a practice.

All mammals with painful injuries should be anaesthetised before any treatment is given, so it is important to find a sympathetic vet from the outset. The Yellow Pages will list all local vets who can be phoned to ask their opinion on working with wildlife casualties.

THE BRITISH VETERINARY ASSOCIATION DOES HAVE A VOLUNTARY DIRECTIVE THAT VETS SHOULD TREAT WILDLIFE CASUALTIES FREE OF CHARGE DURING NORMAL WORKING HOURS. SOME VETS CONFORM, SOME DON'T, BUT IT'S WORTH ASKING.

CLINICAL EXAMINATION

The answers to the previous questions will provide a lead as to the main cause for concern, but any one of these conditions could mask other problems, notably leg abscesses may overlie simple or compound fractures. Check every part of the animal, although with a very lively mammal it may be necessary to wait for 24 hours until it can be anaesthetised or sedated. However, before this course is taken it should be possible, from your remote observations, to give the vet some idea of the major injuries so that the clinical examination could be coupled with any surgical intervention.

A check chart could be kept for each animal with the following information added as a further aid to diagnosis and treatment:

ACTION

Weight   Weighing the animal is essential to calculate the dose rate and monitor progress. Larger animals like badgers, foxes, otters etc. can be weighed in their carrying baskets, the tare weight of which is then deducted. Unfortunately, adult deer and seals are nigh on impossible to weigh, so a good guess based on accepted norms is all we can offer.

Normal weight for adult deer

Muntjac	8–11kg
Chinese water deer	10–14kg
Roe deer	17–25kg
Fallow deer	35–70kg
Sika deer	45–85kg
Red deer	105–180kg

(From Nature Conservancy Council Manual, *The Capture and Handling of Deer*)

Normal weight for adult seals

Common or harbour seal	45–87.5kg females
	55–105kg males
Grey seal	105–186kg females
	170–310kg males

(From Corbet & Southern, *The Handbook of British Mammals*)

Legs   Look and feel along each leg for fractures, dislocations or swellings which may be abscesses (see Ch. 8, pp. 176–8). Pinch the toes to assess if there is any response in the alert animal. Manipulate and push each leg to ensure there is no dislocation at the shoulder or hip. Fold each joint to check any lack of mobility, which may be due to infection or arthritis.

Pelvis   From the rear of the animal manipulate both back legs into the pelvis. Palpate the pelvis – any crepitus (feeling of grating) could mean a fracture or dislocation (see Ch. 8, pp. 181–2, 184).

Spine   Any paralysis of the back legs could point to a spinal injury. Pinching the toes or tail with no response could indicate a broken back. Take particular care and use a stretcher just in case the spinal cord is not yet damaged.

Tail   Check the tail for fractures. Paralysis could be caused by spinal damage.

Feet   Claws, or hooves in a deer, may need clipping. Look for foreign bodies in between the toes and abscesses (see Ch. 8, pp. 176–8) at the roots of the claws or nails.

Mouth   Open the mouth, or lift the lips, to make sure the membranes are moist and pink. Look for damage to the tongue, which could have been bitten in any accident.

Teeth may be broken, infected or have a build-up of calculus (a suppurating smell usually accompanies dental problems). Any injury to the nose may have led to a damaged palate.

Palpate the bottom jaw, feeling for crepitus that may mean a fracture or dislocation (see Ch. 8, pp. 183, 184).

Nose   Clear any exudate from around the nose and feel for the crepitus of a fractured upper jaw. Re-check the palate for damage.

Eyes   The eyes should be clean and bright and respond to light, with the pupils opening and closing. Any deviation points to concussion (see pp. 147–8). Dry or infected eyes should be treated with one of the ophthalmic preparations. Any damage should be seen immediately by a vet. Dirt or other contamination may be bathed out with warm 0.9% saline solution.

Rapid vibration of the eyes, nystagmus, could point to concussion or brain damage.

Ears   Look in the ears for blockages or discharge, possibly caused by ear mites. Bleeding could be the result of a concussive injury.

Fur   The fur should be sleek and well groomed. Any lesions or baldness could be the result of ectoparasites, ringworm or zinc deficiency.

Skin   The skin should feel loose and pliable. Pinch it up into a tent. If it is tight or does not flatten immediately there is some degree of dehydration (see Ch. 6, p. 132).

Bladder   In paralysed animals, feel the abdomen for the bladder. If it feels strained and full there is a risk of kidney failure. It must be emptied! (see pp. 146–7).

Hips   There should be a good spread of fat and muscle across the rump. A very bony animal is thin and not eating because of infection or injury. Look at why it has not been feeding.

Anus   Check the anus is clean and not blocked by over-full anal glands.

Penis   The penis should be withdrawn and out of sight. Paraphimosis is a condition where the penis will not withdraw. It can be subject to infection if not corrected (see p. 163).

Pregnancy   Palpate any female at the time of the year when that species might be expected to be pregnant to try to ascertain if she is pregnant or not. Squeeze the nipples to establish if there is any milk present and if she is therefore likely to be pregnant or a nursing mother.

SPECIFIC CONDITIONS

After this detailed examination, more specific problems may have come to light. General conditions like skin wounds and fractures are dealt with in Chapter 8. The following are some of the common though isolated incidents seen in wild mammal casualties, especially those seen at the Wildlife Hospital Trust.

Abnormalities

Unfortunately some mammals are born with deformities. Most will perish before they leave the nest but some do survive to make it into the adolescent outside world where they find it hard to cope. Sometimes if there is a leg or head deformity, the disability is quite obvious, but other conditions may affect the brain giving abnormal behaviour patterns. The most common example that springs to mind is an **intention tremor**, where a young animal seems to deliberate and hesitate over every step. If there is too much distress then the unfortunate animal may be able to settle into captivity, especially with other permanent residents of the same species. Most often the victim is quite young and *will* settle, becoming quite tame and leading a full life in captivity, although they may not have long life expectancy.

Abrasions

Most animals involved in car accidents do receive grazes and abrasions where the skin is not actually broken. They still need cleaning and treating as a skin wound but should not need antibiotics.

Firstly, the fur, hair or spines around the abrasion have to be cut back. Electric dog clippers are ideal, but if these are not available curved scissors make cutting the fur much easier. Electric clippers will be damaged by hedgehog spines – curved scissors are, unfortunately, the laborious solution for cutting them back to skin level.

Wash the abrasions with a dilute solution of Savlon or Hibiscrub (see Ch. 2, p. 47). If you have a regular intake of animal casualties you would benefit from a Water Pik – a dental tool that pumps disinfectant solution, effectively irrigating away dirt or grit caught in the wound.

Once clean, the abrasions can be covered with Scherisorb Gel (Smith & Nephew), from any chemist, and need no further treatment.

Abscesses (see Ch. 8, pp. 176–8)

Bladder

The bladder is the unsung hero of the anatomy. It collects the urine, the waste material excreted by the kidneys. It expresses the urine out through the urethra on the impulse of various nerves. Failure of these nerves causes the bladder to disfunction and eventually, when overfull, backs urine up to the kidneys leading to uraemia – an abnormally high concentration of urea in the blood, which is an often fatal condition.

Situated centrally between the stomach and the tail, the bladder should always be palpated in animals with any form of paralysis, back damage, pelvic injury or if it is a recently born orphan.

Orphans will need to be stimulated to urinate with a damp cotton bud, whereas adult animals must have their bladders emptied either by gentle pressure on both sides of it, gently pressing towards the tail, or else via an inserted catheter. In both instances these are standard veterinary procedures.

A NON-FUNCTIONING BLADDER SHOULD BE EMPTIED TWICE DAILY OR ELSE THE ANIMAL MAY DIE. THIS IS AN ABSOLUTELY ESSENTIAL LIFE SAVING PROCEDURE AND SHOULD BE LEARNED BY ANYBODY DEALING WITH INJURED MAMMALS.

Burns and scalds

Burns are caused by dry heat whereas scalds are caused by moist heat, e.g. burning fat or chemicals. Treatment for both is very similar, but the degree of pain the animal is suffering must be taken into account before any treatment is given.

Superficial burns which do not break through the skin but affect only the outer one or two layers are extremely painful, whereas **deep burns** that have destroyed the skin have also destroyed the nerve endings, so there is little if any pain.

Burn wounds are sterile because the heat has killed all the skin bacteria. Clip away any fur or hair around the wound site and flush it with sterile 0.9% saline solution to remove any loose debris. Superficial burns may well heal without any further intervention, but deep burn wounds should be covered with sterile paraffin tulle, available from chemists, dressing and referred to the vet. There will be a loss of body fluids which will need to be replaced (see Ch. 6, pp. 132–6).

Scalds and **chemical burns** should be flushed for some time under cold running water and, as in all burn cases, the animal should be kept warm (not under a direct heat source as this causes more pain).

All animals that have been exposed to fire should have their lungs treated by giving antibiotic and corticosteroid courses. That is to say, all burn cases should be referred to the vet.

Concussion

Concussion will usually follow any severe blow to the head of an animal. It may also involve brain damage. The obvious signs are, initially, unconsciousness followed by a lack of co-ordination and lack of normal responses – for example, reduced pupillary reaction to a light source. Any animal with a suspected concussion injury should be given corticosteroids (e.g. dexamethasone) together with antibiotics. Warmth will help the circulation keep flowing and reduce the chance of blood clots forming in the skull.

A head injury may take a considerable time to recede. In fact, a damaged brain cannot regenerate, but the animal may well learn to cope with any disability this may cause. It's rather like a human patient learning to cope after a stroke. Other symptoms may include a tendency of the animal to hold its head towards one shoulder as though it has a stiff neck. Given time, and if they are clearly improving, many concussed animals will be able to be released.

Diarrhoea

Diarrhoea can be a killer if it's not counteracted immediately. Apart from infection that may be causing it, the primary concern is the loss of body fluids. In view of this, any animal with diarrhoea should have its food withheld for 24 hours but it should be given fluids, either Lectade or International Rehydrating Fluid, by mouth or Hartmanns by intravenous infusion (see Ch. 6, pp. 134–6). The minimum amount offered should be 50ml per kg of body weight per day.

Information that will be useful to the vet is:
a) how often the diarrhoea occurs
b) its colour and smell
c) any evidence of straining
d) the presence of blood, worms or mucus.

Dislocations (see Ch. 8, p. 184)

Ear problems

The ears of mammals often cause problems. Common problems in wild mammals are **ear mites**, **ear infections** and **maggots**.

Many species suffer from ear mites, which can be identified with an aurioscope. Many acaricidal ear drops are available that will clear the problem with regular applications. A vet will advise and prescribe the most suitable preparation – for instance, GAC Ear Drops (Arnolds) or Oterna Ear Drops (Coopers Pitman-Moore). Evidence of mites is really best confirmed with the microscope, but some evidence may be seen with an aurioscope that facilitates looking deep into the ear.

Ear infections usually show themselves as a purulent discharge. Your vet will prescribe one of the topical aural preparations – usually drops containing antibiotics.

All **maggots** should be removed and the ear flushed with dilute Hibiscrub just to make sure. Ear preparations containing Gamma-BHC, like GAC drops from a vet, will also encourage maggots to evacuate. However, check any maggot-ridden ear at least twice a day in case just one maggot has escaped your attention.

Endoparasites

I think it can safely be assumed that most wild mammals have some form of endoparasite. In most cases, the parasite load has little effect on the host animal but, to give any casualty the best chances of recovery and post-release survival, **worming** should become a normal procedure. Proprietary wormers like those sold for dogs and cats are effective for **roundworms** but may miss other forms especially, for instance, **lung-worms**, which seem to affect most hedgehogs.

Two injections of ivermectin given three weeks apart will remove most species. However, in hedgehogs, ivermectin injections should be accompanied by an injection of dexamethasone to help the lungs to clear, so a vet is needed to give directions.

Incidentally, ivermectin can be given either by injection or by mouth. It is very unstable, but can be mixed 1:9 with propylene glycol, enabling it to be kept mixed for up to 30 days. It is toxic to some dogs but appears to be ideal for wild animals, where it can also assist by removing ectoparasites like mange mites.

Generally, **tapeworms** are not going to pose any problem so, in the main, specific treatments against these are not necessary.

Euthanasia

I am completely opposed to euthanasia unless the animal cannot possibly maintain itself, even in captivity. The so-called 'putting an animal out of its misery' is just a ploy in many cases because somebody cannot be bothered to care for the animal until it recovers.

There are so many sophisticated drugs available these days that any animal being treated need not suffer pain or psychological discomfort while it is in care. The use of analgesics, like Finadyne or Temgesic from a vet, have been shown to enhance the chances of recovery.

Bearing this in mind, it's worthwhile assessing a casualty as though it were a human being. Would any of us give up on a human patient just because he or she was temporarily uncomfortable and stressed?

Of course, there are situations where euthanasia should be the only answer; even then each candidate should be assessed and re-assessed with the vet. A VET IS REALLY THE ONLY PERSON TRAINED SUFFICIENTLY TO SAY WHETHER AN ANIMAL NEEDS TO BE KILLED. But even then, question the prognosis and try, just one more time, to see if between you an answer can be found.

In my opinion, mammal euthanasia is most humane by intravenous injection, when the animal just appears to fall asleep with no discomfort. I know that sometimes an injection is given directly into the heart or liver. I feel that this is cruel and should never be allowed to happen. In fact, with any euthanasia I always insist that the patient is anaesthetised first. Thankfully we meet very few hopeless cases and do not have to make this final decision.

Typical cases where there is no hope are:
Any mammal that has lost two or more legs.
An animal with a break in the spinal cord – a broken back should be X-rayed to establish the extent of the damage.
An animal with no bottom jaw.
An animal paralysed with no sign of improvement after a week or so. And unfortunately, for safety's sake, any animal with a disease contagious to humans, like leptospirosis and, of course, rabies. The vet will advise on diagnosis.

Euthanasia is final so never ever treat it, like some people do, as a matter-of-fact routine: there could always be an answer.

Eyes
We all know how tender our eyes can be and it's the same with the eyes of wild mammals. They are essential for survival and painful if injured. ANY EYE DAMAGE WHATSOEVER SHOULD BE REFERRED TO A VET EXPERIENCED IN EYE PROBLEMS. However, first-aid measures can be taken both to relieve any discomfort and possibly save the eye.

The only preparations put into the eyes should be those specifically designed for animals' eyes. However, bathing an eye in warm clean water or warmed saline solution can help flush out any debris or in the summer fly eggs or maggots.

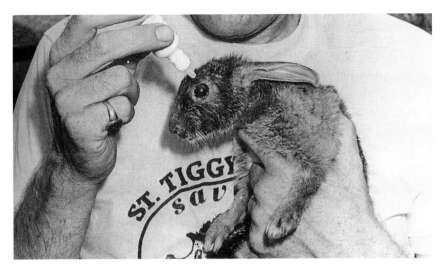

Only ever use eye drops prepared especially for mammals

Saline solution

1 heaped teaspoon table salt in 1 quart boiling water, allowed to cool.

Any eye injury can be safely lubricated with bland chloramphenicol eye ointment, from a vet, spread along the bottom eyelid. Never use, without veterinary advice, any eye ointment containing any form of steroid as it may impede healing.

It is essential that an animal can close its eyes or the eye may dry out. An unconscious animal or one with an eye injury may not be able to close its eye, which must then be lubricated several times a day with hypromellose drops or once daily with Lacri-Lube, an ocular lubricant available at most chemists.

Veterinary attention is essential with all suspected eye damage or any infection may travel along the optic nerve directly into the brain.

In **myxomatosis** (see pp. 159–60), a rabbit's eyelids become swollen, inflamed and infected. Bathing them apart with warmed saline may bring some relief and in the remote instance when a rabbit survives the disease, keeping the eyelids open will prevent them healing together.

A constant flickering of the eyeball, known as **nystagmus**, could be a sign of concussion (see pp. 147–8).

Quite often, especially as the result of a road accident, the eyeball may be pushed out from its socket. Lubricating it with Lacri-Lube and pushing it back into the socket may well save it. If not, the vet may have to remove it completely.

The loss of one eye is not a great hindrance to most species, with some even surviving in captivity well with no eyes. Mammals have a good sense of smell and can usually find their food and partners without necessarily having to see perfectly. For instance, blind seals cope very well. But think twice about releasing the following species:

a) All other species with total blindness, e.g.:

i) nocturnal animals, which may mistake the time of day

ii) animals which rely on sight such as deer or rabbits – they may miss a predator

iii) jumping animals – squirrels and dormice – which will misjudge leaps.

b) Male deer with one eye lost – it will be at a disadvantage fighting during the rut.

c) Squirrels with one eye lost – they will not be able to judge jumps.

Fly strike (myiasis)

During the warmer months of the year invasion by **fly larvae (maggots)** is one of the commonest life-threatening afflictions of wildlife casualties. Untreated, the maggots will eventually kill the animal in a slow and agonising attack.

The first signs are the fly eggs themselves laid on any unmoving tissue, whether the tissue is dead or alive. Any unmoving animal is likely to be attacked. The eggs themselves are small, cigar shaped and white, laid in clusters and fixed by a form of adhesion making them difficult to remove.

However they *must* all be laboriously picked off with forceps or brushed off with a stiff brush (I use a washing-up brush on the fur or spines specifically for this purpose).

The main victims are **hedgehogs**; many are found with eggs in and around the eyes, over the head and in the ears and mouth, along the skirt, where the spines meet the furry underneath, and around the base of the tail. The eggs hatch into tiny maggots within hours and then become a major problem that moves. Clipping the fur (see p. 146) will remove many, but any residue will to be removed by hand with forceps.

Once they have hatched, the maggots seek out warm, damp places like wounds, ears, eyes, mouth, under the legs and in the genital area. They have to be picked off or flushed out with dilute Savlon. Insecticide powders seem to have no effect whatsoever. Maggots deep in the ears will evacuate if the ears are flushed with an ear preparation containing Gamma-BHC. GAC Drops are suitable and available from a vet.

Maggots do like damp areas and will perish if they dry out, so warm-drying any infestation with a hair drier does have some effect. The animal may be unhappy about this but the warming will settle it and, of course, the maggots *must* be removed.

Farmers use Battle Fly and Maggot Paste to cope with maggots. A strong yellow ointment, it is packed into an affected wound and removed, as a plug, after 24 hours when all the maggots will have been killed. All dead maggots in a wound should be removed manually. I hear stories of animals being 'put out of their misery' just because they are suffering from fly strike. This is totally unnecessary and most will recover if given patience and treatment.

Foot problems

Hedgehogs may be found with a foot extremely swollen and painful. There is invariably some infection and maybe fractures present (see Ch. 8, pp. 180–1). Any mass of infected material should be lanced and cleaned out and a course of antibiotics instituted. Your vet may wish to carry out a sensitivity test on the infected material before prescribing a particular antibiotic.

Hedgehogs also have a habit of chewing painful or infected feet. Their fellow hedgehogs may even do it for them. The bitter sprays available at pet shops have some effect, but we find the most effective deterrent to be a lady's cylindrical plastic hair curler slid over the leg and held at its top by a strip of adhesive plaster. The lattice-work of the curler allows air to get to the foot, whereas enclosing it in a dressing may exacerbate any infection.

Bitten-off toes can be cleaned with Dermisol Multi-cleanse Solution (Smith-Kline Beecham) coupled with antibiotic cover, supplied by a vet. As long as there are still some pads left on the bottom of the foot the hedgehog will manage quite adequately. Hedgehogs and badgers have very long claws by nature, but if a foot is out of contact with the ground through injury the claws may grow too long and need clipping. Dog toe-nail clippers, available at pet shops, are ideal.

Similar, **deer hooves** are kept trim by constant use but may overgrow because of an injury. They will need paring with a hoof knife. Any hoof, nail or claw has a blood supply to its cuticle. Cutting too short may produce bleeding, which can be stemmed with a caustic or styptic pencil from the chemists, but is best avoided.

A muntjac we rescued from a walled electricity substation had, in its efforts to escape, worn its hooves away completely. It did grow new ones but because their bony centres did not regenerate the hooves were hollow and the deer could not be released. It is now living almost free-range in captivity.

ANY ANIMAL THAT COMPLETELY LOSES TWO FEET CANNOT CONTINUE AS THE LEG STUMPS ARE NOT SUFFICIENT TO CARRY THE ANIMAL. THIS TYPE OF DISABILITY SHOULD BE REFERRED TO THE VET FOR EUTHANASIA.

Fractures (see Ch. 8, pp. 178–84)

Haemorrhage (bleeding)
An animal suffering a **severe haemorrhage** because of an accident is probably not going to live long enough to reach a care facility. Emergency, on-the-spot, first aid can be attempted by applying a pressure pad to a wound or applying a tourniquet to a limb (release every 10 minutes) and rushing a casualty to the nearest veterinary centre.

Unfortunately, no direct blood replacements are available for wild animals, but if blood loss is not great a plasma substitute like Haemaccel may help restore the circulating blood volume lost.

Away from the accident site and in more antiseptic conditions, fractured blood vessels can be held with artery forceps and referred to the vet for ligature with absorbable catgut.

Small seepages of blood, especially from nails, can sometimes be stemmed with a dusting of wound powder. More persistent bleeding may need cauterising with a caustic pencil. Bleeding from the nose will stop after a short while, but blood may block the nostrils, which can be wiped clear with a cotton bud dipped in dilute Savlon (see Ch. 2, p. 47).

Bleeding from the anus, vulva or penis should be referred to the vet for diagnosis as, respectively, the problems could range from enteritis to cystitis, or even be the result of traumatic injury.

Head damage (see also, Concussion, above)

Apart from the internal effects of concussion, some head injuries, especially in hedgehogs, seem particularly severe, with massive skin loss and fractures to the nasal bones. The **fractures** will have to be left to **heal spontaneously**, but the **skin wounds** can be cleaned up and **sutured** as best as possible (see Ch. 8, pp. 173–5). In order to keep the casualty breathing cleanly, sterile plastic tubes can be inserted under the sutured skin as temporary nostrils. Whenever there is damage to the snout also check inside the mouth for injuries to the palate. These can usually be sutured.

During treatment for **nasal injuries** the nose mucus may itself cause breathing difficulties. Injections with Bisolvon (Boehringer Ingelheim) will loosen any nasal material to bring relief and can be prescribed by a vet. Actual damage to the skull surrounding the brain must be referred to a specialist veterinary surgeon.

Abscesses on the scalp and face can be lanced, drained and cleaned just like abscesses on other parts of the body (see Ch. 8, pp. 176–8).

Hyperthermia (over-heating)

This is the condition that kills dogs locked in cars on hot or even just warm days. It does happen to wild mammals, especially if they are, for one reason or another, unable to get out of direct sunlight. Dehydration (see Ch. 6, pp. 132–4) is a common cause of overheating in wild animals, especially those being transported in warm vehicles.

When the critical body temperature is exceeded, the depression of the central nervous system brings about death by respiratory failure. It's often not possible to take a wild mammal's temperature so visual symptoms are the trigger to take urgent action. Lying flat out and panting, often audibly, with the tongue extended, just like a hot dog, are sure signs the animal is feeling the heat.

It may sound drastic but the most immediate relief can be obtained by **immersing the animal in cold water**, keeping the head above water, or, as I did when meeting a very hot badger which would have still have been dangerous to handle, pour buckets of cold water over it. If it's

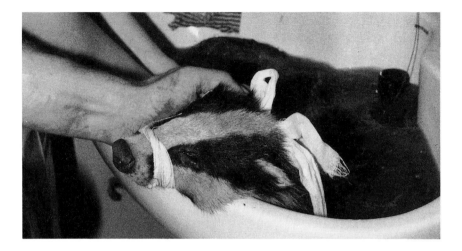

Always bind a badger's jaws when treating it – it has the most powerful bite of any British mammal

going to work then the recovery is rapid; if not, a vet should be called who can try aspirin or chlorpromazine to relieve the condition.

Hypothermia

The opposite of hyperthermia, hypothermia occurs when an animal's temperature falls below its normal range. An animal that is unconscious or a very young animal will be unable to shiver and maintain some sort of body heat. On touching the animal it will feel cold. A slow warm-up is best, but initially it should be **wrapped in blankets** or a space blanket before warmed intravenous fluids can be administered.

Patients recovering after a general anaesthetic are subject to chilling and should be kept warm either in a **hospital cage** or wrapped in insulating material such as **bubble wrap** packing material.

The use of heated pads is not recommended as a comatose or unconscious patient will not be able to move away from too much heat. Take particular care when releasing an animal that has been shaved for treatment. Any bald patches may make the animal susceptible to cold during the winter months and colder nights. DON'T RELEASE THEM UNTIL THEY CAN MAINTAIN HEAT NORMALLY.

Leptospirosis

Knows as Weil's disease in humans, leptospirosis is rare in wildlife casualties *but can be fatal to man* if contracted and not treated early enough. The well-know brown rat, of plague proportions these days, is the main vector, with a large proportion of their population carrying the disease, which is passed on via their urine. DO NOT, FOR THIS REASON, HANDLE RAT CASUALTIES.

Any animal I take in with even a slight yellowing of its skin or mucous membranes is treated with caution and **isolation**. It is only handled if necessary, with rubber gloves, and is referred to a vet immediately for diagnosis. To protect staff and volunteers we make no attempt to treat leptospirosis, although it can be done with very strict isolation and barrier nursing.

The yellowing of the jaundiced tissue is one sign, a heavy thirst and bleeding from the nose with no history of trauma could also signify the disease.

TAKE NO CHANCES – REFER ANY SUSPECTED CASE TO THE VET AND MAKE SURE THAT YOUR DOG'S VACCINATIONS ARE UP TO DATE.

Lice
Lice are flat, wingless insects which have a terrible stigma attached to them when they are found on humans. However, most wild mammals, except perhaps hedgehogs and foxes, seem to have their quota, which live symbiotically with their host. Lice, though, can be carriers of disease and any animal handled would benefit from a dusting of a pyrethrum-based insect powder.

Lice are host-specific and one species of lice will not leave its host species to live on another, not even a human one.

Loss of balance
Any animal that is weak, emaciated or dehydrated may not be able to stand, but lack of balance will have an underlying cause that is giving rise to the weakness or emaciation. True loss of balance or equilibrium is invariably caused by a head or ear problem (see pp. 147–8, 148–9).

A **head injury** is usually the result of an accident and can be treated with corticosteroids like dexamethasone. *Otitis interna* is damage to the delicate organs of balance inside the ear. Symptoms include loss of balance and often a tilting of the head. The condition may be a result of infection spreading through the ear which can usually be countered by routine antibiotic therapy by injection.

Maggots (see Fly strike, pp. 152–3)

Mange and Mange Mites

Mites are microscopic members of the Arachnida, which includes spiders, ticks and scorpions. Minute though they are, mites still cause serious problems to wild mammals who are unfortunate enough to be afflicted by them.

Only really visible under a microscope, any scabby or crusty skin lesions or, in hedgehogs, a powdery exudate around the face and ear, could well be mite infestation. A vet with laboratory facilities can take a skin scraping to confirm the mite's presence. The skin scraping will need to be softened in clearing fluid (10% potassium hydroxide solution) before putting under the microscope. The two species most often affected are **foxes** and **hedgehogs**, both of which can be treated with ivermectin injections. Even the most debilitated fox will recover, given the right treatment and support, from the ravages of the sarcoptic mange – a condition many people will have you believe is untreatable.

Ivermectin can also be administered by mouth, so if a fox visits you regularly, it can have its weight estimated and be offered food laced with a calculated dose. It will need to be repeated after three weeks to be fully effective. However, if there is more than one fox visiting there could be a danger of one taking both doses. In this situation, a cage trap may be the answer to catch the target fox and release it after treatment. Remember, ivermectin can cause problems to some dogs, so they should not be allowed near the bait.

(Incidentally, I am allergic to sarcoptic manage and always try to wear protective gloves when handling an affected fox. The mass of spots that erupt on my skin within hours are not mange but merely an allergy, which is usually brought under control by antihistamine tablets.)

Ear mites (see Ear problems, pp. 148–9)

Mouth disorders (see also Teeth, pp. 168–70)

Almost any mammal will resent anybody looking into its mouth and will need some form of anaesthesia for an inspection or treatment to take place. Teeth, in particular, can be a major problem.

Other problems, especially after collision accidents, are **damage to**

the tongue, **palate** and **lips**. The tongue is often caught on a tooth and should be lifted clear with forceps. Lacerations can be sutured but this must be carried out, under anaesthetic, by a vet.

Tongues are sometimes infected, especially in hedgehogs. As yet there appears to be no routine recommended antibiotic and each vet will have his or her own opinion. Swollen tongues could be infection or an insect sting. Antibiotics and antihistamine may bring relief and if the condition is life-threatening then corticosteroids can be used.

Torn palates and **torn lips** can be sutured by the vet.

Always check inside a suspect mouth for foreign bodies. I have removed a piece of lamb bone jamming a hedgehog's mouth, hedgehog spines spiked into the palate of other animals, and all manner of pieces of string, line and wire, which are beds for infection in the soft tissue inside animals' mouths.

Myxomatosis

Myxomatosis is a disease that can break your heart. Man introduced it and continues to encourage it, yet I am sure that if the perpetrators of this horror saw the animals I have to deal with, and if they are in the slightest bit human, they would have nightmares about the pain and suffering they are causing.

Myxomatosis kills slowly and painfully – and there is no cure

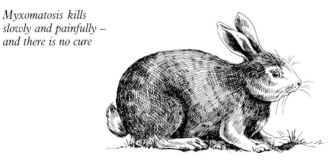

Tiny bunnies are brought into me never having been able to see, for as soon as their eyes opened the infection of myxomatosis sealed their eyelids again for ever. The disease takes no account of age and ravages young and old alike, taking up to 19 days to strangle every organ in the poor rabbit's body slowly until death ensues.

During the early stage of the illness, however, the rabbits will continue to feed and breed as if nothing is happening until, finally, their inability to see and breathe properly slows them down so much that starvation takes over.

Any rabbit brought to us, sick or not, is isolated immediately and powdered with flea powder. It is the fleas that are the main carriers of the disease from rabbit to rabbit and must be prevented from escaping onto other rabbits.

We must be grateful myxomatosis only affects rabbits, although there have been some cases confirmed in hares. All other species, including humans, are not affected by the disease. All carrying boxes and bedding should be burnt after use by a diseased rabbit.

The first noticeable symptoms of myxomatosis are swelling of the eyelids, which become sealed, followed by swelling of the nose and genitalia.

The first thing to consider is that this common symptom of infected eyes may simply be due to severe conjunctivitis. Cleaning the eyes with warmed saline solution (see p. 151) and then treating with plain chloramphenicol ointment may bring relief.

Some rabbits will overcome myxomatosis themselves but it has to be via their own natural resilience because it is caused by a virus, and as such there is no cure we can provide. There is great controversy about whether the afflicted animal should even be kept alive. I only wish some of the scientists, who were so quick to find a treatment for parvovirus in dogs and mobillivirus in scals, would set their minds to trying to bring some relief for rabbits suffering from myxomatosis.

As I said, some rabbits will recover, but you must always ask yourself whether the animal is suffering pointlessly by being kept alive.

Captive rabbits can be protected for nine months with a vaccine. However, the vaccine is very unstable when mixed so many rabbits will need to be vaccinated at the same time to avoid wasting serum.

Oil

Animals do get affected by oil but not on the same scale as birds. Treatment can be along the same lines as for oiled birds.

There are now established methods, developed from treatment of the oiled sea otters stranded in the *Exxon Valdez* spill in Alaska. If any

British otters or seals are caught in an oil spill, they should really be referred to a specialist centre.

Basically, the affected animal should be thoroughly bathed in a 2% solution of Fairy Liquid at 45°C. Afterwards, rinse and keep the animal warm until it is completely dry.

Orphans

The rearing of orphaned mammals is far too involved and complex to deal with in this book. However, we at St Tiggywinkles are always willing to advise on any orphaned mammal problem and have some fact sheets available if a stamped addressed envelope is sent in.

There are certain questions that should always be asked before 'rescuing' an apparently abandoned youngster. Many mammal mothers leave their youngsters unattended for long periods and will return to feed them at regular intervals. Sometimes people pick these apparent orphans up thinking they are abandoned when, in fact, they are not. It used to be thought that because of the human scent on them, these rescued youngsters could not be returned. In fact, some can. If the youngster is **put back exactly where it was found**, the parent will eventually come back and claim its truants.

As always with wildlife, there are no hard and fast rules about dealing with orphans, and different species require various solutions. Some solutions to the problem are suggested below:

Deer are the most common 'orphans' – youngsters are left alone in long grass for many hours every day. Rescued fawns can still be returned after 48 hours.

Foxes – a rescued youngster may have strayed from the den or been lost *en route*. On returning it to the site where it was found and watching from a distance, the vixen will usually be seen to round it up and take it to rejoin the family. Of course, if she does not return at all then the cub will need to be rescued and reared.

Badgers – badger cubs do not normally roam far from the sett. Any badger cub found out and alone well away from a sett therefore needs rescuing. It is inadvisable to put it into a sett you may come across because if it's the wrong one, the cub may be attacked.

Hedgehogs – any hedgehog nest uncovered accidentally should be recovered immediately and left undisturbed. The babies should not be touched. The female hedgehog (the male takes no part in family life) may well not spend much time at the nest and could sleep elsewhere. She will not normally abandon her offspring.

However, any youngsters found away from the nest will need rescuing. It is not advisable to put a stray youngster into a nest as it may be killed by the returning female.

During the winter months any hedgehog weighing less than 600g may well not survive hibernation. These are usually late-bred juveniles that should be taken into care until the following spring.

Seals – just like deer, the adult female will leave her pup alone for many hours at a time. It should not be rescued unless it is very obviously sick or injured.

Squirrels – young squirrels often fall from their nest tree, but it is usually futile to try to return them to their nursery. If they can be picked up, they need rescuing.

Mice – a mouse nest may easily be uncovered in compost or rubbish heap. Leave it alone and cover it up again and the mother, who will have fled, will return when you have left.

Hares – leverets are left hidden in long grass by their mothers. They do not need rescuing and should be left alone or returned if they have been picked up.

Rabbits – any baby rabbit out in the open which can be picked up needs rescuing.

Bats – baby bats, no larger than a fingernail, are often found clinging to walls and curtains. It's often not practical to try to reunite them with their nursery colony so they, too, will need rescuing. Remember, though, that an adult pipistrelle is also very tiny and should not be confused with a youngster.

These brief notes cover the more regular incidents of apparent orphans which, in the majority of cases, should be left alone. However, any young animal that is injured or caught by a dog or cat should be taken in for medical attention.

Penis

Injuries to the penis can cause not only severe haemorrhaging but can block the exit of urine from the bladder, leading to further complications (see pp. 146–7). Any injury should be **referred to the vet** for treatment.

Other conditions that occur regularly are **paraphimosis** (where the penis will not slide back into the prepuce, the sheath of skin usually protruding from the abdomen), infection or abscesses on the penis (which should be referred to the vet) and, during the summer, the invasion of the prepuce by maggots (see pp. 152–3). The latter is always worth looking for in hedgehogs.

Obviously any **maggots** should be removed and the prepuce flushed with antiseptic, whether dilute Savlon or Hibiscrub (see Ch. 2, p. 47).

Paraphimosis is serious but can sometimes be rectified by the application of cold water or ice to the penis or temporarily restricting the blood flow just in front of the scrotum (not present in a hedgehog). If the condition continues then the animal must be referred to the vet.

In groups of young, suckling animals there is sometimes damage to the penis by other members of the nursery. Watch for signs of it and, if necessary, apply a bitter spray to prevent further occurrences.

Poisons

There is very little we can do to help a wild animal that has been poisoned – we cannot be sure from its symptoms that it *has* been poisoned and, in most cases, could not identify the poison anyway.

There is often excess salivation accompanied by convulsions, which the layman would generally describe as a 'fit'. However, the same symptoms can be caused by other types of illness, so they might be the result of poisoning or something else such as epilepsy.

The more common poisons likely to be encountered in wild mammal casualties are either accidental – like poisoning with rat or slug bait – or intentional, where poisoned meat is illegally put out to trap raptors and predators.

Squirrels are often affected intentionally with **Warfarin** or **Difenacoum**, rat baits that interfere with blood clotting agents. Affected animals suffer spontaneous internal haemorrhages, seen externally as pale or bleeding gums. Vitamin K can be injected by a vet as an antidote and the animal kept quiet so as not to induce any further bleeding.

Metaldehyde poisoning from eating **slug pellets** is very common. I only wish people would stop using these as they are killers of all forms of animal. Symptoms include convulsions and salivation coupled with what I call hypersensitivity, where an animal nearly 'jumps out of its skin' if you merely click your fingers. There is no antidote, although sedatives will calm the animal, which is probably going to die.

That is the story with poisons – the animal is **probably going to die**. To my mind, as there is no cure, prevention is the only answer. If only people would realise that flea sprays, slug pellets, weedkillers, insecticides and some wood preservatives *do* kill, then perhaps they would stop using them. For instance, many more hedgehogs would be saved if people, especially vets, did not spray them with aerosol flea sprays, which contain some of the more deadly poisons like dichlorvos. Read the small print and see for yourself.

Premature birth

Unfortunately, some animals are injured while they are pregnant, which can lead to abortion, with all the subsequent complications. This can happen at any time of the year with some species, although others have specific months when they might give birth. For instance, badgers are more than likely to give birth in February or March, whereas muntjac deer will have youngsters in any month of the year.

All female casualties should be checked and if there is a suspicion of pregnancy or abortion then they should be examined by the vet. This is particularly important in cases of suspected pelvic damage.

Rabies

At the moment rabies is rarely present in Britain. It can occur, however, so anybody likely to be picking up a wild mammal casualty should consult their doctor for a pre-exposure rabies vaccination. It's not the old wives' tale of injection into the stomach, but a simple inoculation just like any other.

The mad-dog syndrome is not always the classic symptom, either – many rabies cases display the 'dumb' form of the disease, which manifests itself in a flaccid paralysis, drooling saliva and other signs, none of which would make anybody think the animal was suffering from the virus. IF THERE IS ANY DOUBT, HANDLE THE ANIMAL VERY, VERY CAREFULLY, CONFINE IT SECURELY AND CONTACT THE VET IMMEDIATELY.

If rabies does come into Britain then I am more afraid of people's reaction than of the disease itself. There are well-controlled contingency plans to deal with an outbreak but it worries me that anybody with a shotgun will be out shooting everything that moves.

There are oral vaccines against rabies that have been used very successfully in many other countries, especially with foxes. Perhaps we should start vaccinating our wildlife now before the panic sets in.

Respiratory problems

The treatment of respiratory problems is very much the domain of the veterinary surgeon, but it's vital to be aware of likely incidence so that urgent remedial action can be instigated.

Hedgehogs are likely to be infested with **lungworm**, which can predispose to pneumonia. If a hedgehog can be seen to be breathing heavily then it needs assessing with a stethoscope and treating. Antibiotics are needed for pneumonia but ivermectin coupled with dexamethasone will shift the inevitable lungworm. Hedgehogs also suffer from **nose injuries** which force them to breathe through their mouths. To help them, any blocking of the nostrils can be cleared away with damp cotton buds and Bisolvon administered in an injection by a vet to relieve the mucus build-up. There may also be damage to the palate which may need suturing (see Ch. 8, pp. 174–5).

Hedgehogs with severe breathing difficulties also benefit from oxygen therapy in a nebuliser and the administration of Millophyline-V or Ventipulmin as respiratory stimulants.

Excess fluid in the lung cavity can be carefully controlled with frusemide (Lasix) but care has to be taken to replace fluids removed from elsewhere in the body.

Squirrels often suffer **nose damage** resulting from falls. Treatment is the same as for hedgehogs.

Badgers, foxes and deer as road casualties often suffer damage to the **chest** resulting in a build-up of fluids. Any road casualty should have its lungs assessed with the help of a stethoscope and, if necessary, any fluid controlled with frusemide.

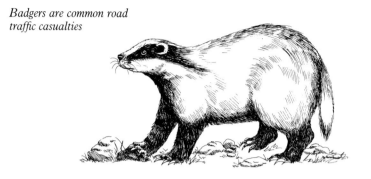

Badgers are common road traffic casualties

Very old animals may suffer from **heart conditions** and fluid build-up in the lungs. These animals should not be released but can do very well on regular medication with frusemide and drugs to treat the heart conditions.

As you can see, all chest problems require drugs of one sort or the other, all of which are the province of the vet, except perhaps for the use of ivermectin for lungworm in hedgehogs, which can be treated as a routine worming procedure.

Ringworm

The only recurring incident of ringworm in wild mammals is in **hedgehogs**. Typical signs are bald patches, flaky skin and the loss of spines. Unlike the ringworm of dogs and cats, hedgehog ringworm, *Trichophyton erinacei*, does not fluoresce under ultra-violet light. The only way of confirming its presence is with a test known as a Fungassay test.

Treatment is with oral medication of Griseofulvin, available from a vet, either as a powder on the food or as a syrup, Fulcin, given by pipette. Both need at least six weeks to be effective.

Ringworm is contagious to humans and appears initially as little raised bumps on the fingers. The application of Canesten ointment usually clears it within a day or two.

Skin problems

Skin problems, other than mange (see p. 158) or ringworm (above), are unusual in wild animals. The only other common occurrence is, once again, in the **hedgehog**, which may be completely or partially bald, yet which has no signs of either mange or ringworm. The cases we have handled appear to be suffering from a deficiency of zinc and respond very quickly, often within a week, to vitamin additives containing a high percentage of zinc, e.g. Vetamin + Zinc (Millpledge).

As a rule, animals with tatty coats will all benefit from the addition of a vitamin supplement to their feed.

Snares or netting

For some inhuman reason some snares are still legal in this country and are set to garrotte. I have had to remove snares from foxes, badgers, deer, rabbits, dogs, cats and even geese. It just shows how indiscriminate snares can be. The so-called free-running snare is legal, with the locking snare being against the law. In practice, however, the free-running snare invariably frays with the efforts of the victim to escape and becomes a locking snare.

Intentional use of locking snares should be reported to the Wildlife Liaison Officer of the Local Police.

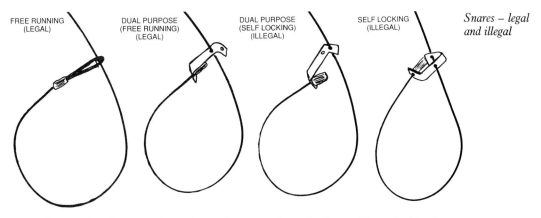

FREE RUNNING (LEGAL) DUAL PURPOSE (FREE RUNNING) (LEGAL) DUAL PURPOSE (SELF LOCKING) (ILLEGAL) SELF LOCKING (ILLEGAL)

Snares – legal and illegal

Any animal trapped under a fence or in a hedge will probably be caught in a snare. Sometimes it is possible to release the snare and the animal but, in my experience, the contusions caused by the snare will not erupt from the skin for a few days. It is always worth holding the animal for at least a week to watch for previously unseen damage.

Snares are not easy to cut but can be chopped up with a good pair of fencing pliers – a must for anybody who walks in the countryside. Look in any well-marked animal runs for snares, then pull them out with the fencing pliers, chop them into little pieces and leave them as a notice to the trapper that you are aware of his practice.

Similarly, but accidentally, animals will get ensnared in netting. Incidences I have dealt with include cricket, tennis, football, bean, chain-link and sea-fishing nets. In most cases the patient must be anaesthetised to make sure that every trace or ligature is removed. Then, once again, it is necessary to observe the animal for a few days, particularly looking out for the animal chewing at the site when any pins and needles occur as a leg or foot regains its blood supply. Bitter sprays available at pet shops or even an Elizabethan collar may be necessary to stop self-mutilation.

Stress

Although not as widespread as in birds, some species of mammal suffer considerably from stress, often resulting in the little understood condition of **post-capture myopathy** that can kill an animal up to two weeks after its confinement.

The most common sufferers in the mammal fraternity are **deer** and **hares**, although **rabbits** and **foxes** may succumb, especially if they have been involved in a long chase.

We counter stress in deer casualties by routinely giving an initial large dose of dexamethasone (e.g. 3ml to a muntjac), as they are taken into care. If they do not settle and threaten to injure themselves, as they often do, they are maintained on diazepam or midazolam, given daily. Results of a new drug in animals, Piportil-Depot, which can sedate a deer for some weeks at a time, have meant that long-term treatments of severe injuries in adult deer can now be undertaken with a high degree of success.

In order to ease the stress that any wild animal must feel if it is taken into care just follow the simple do's and don'ts opposite.

Teeth

Teeth problems are the cause of the natural deaths of many wild mammals. If the animal is lucky, its teeth wear out, making it difficult for the animal to feed in old age. More often, though, infection caused by teeth problems spreads slowly but inexorably, killing the animal which is often in the prime of its life.

Do's and don'ts to avoid stress in mammals

Don't handle the animal unnecessarily
Don't look it straight in the eyes
Don't house it with an aggressive animal
Don't talk or make any loud noises
Don't, or try not to, allow it to sense a predatory species nearby –
    remembering man is a predator

Do cover its cage
Do use red light bulbs for illumination (most mammals are colour
    blind, but red light seems to calm some adult deer)
Do keep it warm but not too hot
Do keep gregarious species with others of its own kind, e.g. deer,
    rabbits, badgers, fox cubs, but watch for aggression.
Do give orphaned mammals a cuddly toy as a surrogate mother.
Do encourage the vet to use diazepam or midazolam to calm an excited
    animal

We now make it a practice to check the teeth of every mammal taken in by the hospital. Any remedial dental work can then be undertaken by a dentist specialising in animals – human dentists do not have the requisite tools to deal with some of the larger animals, whose teeth are a lot harder than ours.

Hedgehogs suffer horrendous mouth problems, which usually start with a mysterious build up of calculus (tartar) on the molar teeth. The calculus causes exposures of the gums, allowing infection to spread into the jaw bone and eventually down the neck and into the chest.

Every vet has a dental descaling unit for use on dogs and cats and can use this to descale a hedgehog's teeth and remove any that are infected or loose. Antibiotic treatment (clindomycin is the most suitable at present), is also vital in order to stem the infection.

Badgers and foxes suffer from fractures and cavities which should be treated by an animal dentist before the creature is released. It's quite a costly procedure, needing not only the dentist but also an experienced veterinary surgeon to maintain sophisticated long-term anaesthesia.

Without treatment, compromised teeth could be painful to the animal, quite apart from the risk of the spread of infection.

Squirrels and other rodents often appear after an accident looking as though their teeth have been knocked out. Owing to the growth pattern of rodent teeth, which is continuous, there is a huge reservoir of tooth left in the gums so, in fact, the teeth have only been broken off and will soon grow again.

The problem with rodent incisors is that they sometimes grow out of control. As they grow, they should be honed down by the opposing incisors, but they sometimes miss their opposite number and never wear down. Any animal with this malocclusion should be kept in captivity as its needs its teeth clipping regularly to keep them under control.

Deer. Some species, notably muntjac and Chinese water deer, have sharp tusks in their upper jaw. They can generally move a fraction in their sockets, but if broken should be treated as any other broken tooth and be filled or removed by the dentist.

Skin wounds (see Ch. 8, pp. 172–6)

Ticks

Ticks are members of the Arachnida, like mites. They appear on mammals as small, pin-head sized lumps until they gorge themselves with blood and become about pea-sized.

Unless they are present in their hundreds on an animal I do not regard them as a major problem. In fact, as they are resistant to insecticides and the only way to remove them is by pulling them off, their mouthparts, which could be left in the skin, can be the source of an infection far more damaging than their one-off blood-sucking propensity.

I remove them individually by sliding a pair of fine artery forceps between them and the skin and lifting them clear with a sharp tug. One system recommended to me for the inexperienced tick-lifter is to cover each tick with a wad of cotton wool soaked in anaesthetic ether. The tick is apparently then anaesthetised and easily lifted free. There is also a tick-removing tool available which does seem an ideal way of relieving a difficult situation.

One thing to remember is that ticks, once free of the skin, can walk considerable distances and attach themselves undetected to human and other animals, so make sure that any that are removed are disposed of in a bowl of disinfectant.

In the main, I think the attempts to remove just a few ticks can cause more problems than leaving them where they are.

Tongue

Most problems affecting an animal's tongue are caused during a traumatic accident, when it can be damaged by being caught on teeth. If necessary, the vet may want to suture a serious tear.

Tongue infections occur especially in hedgehogs and can be treated systemically with antibiotics. **Swollen tongues** may be the result of infection or could be caused by an insect sting, in which case anti-histamine may help relieve the symptoms. A swollen tongue can cause suffocation, so should be treated without delay. Ice cubes may bring a temporary relief.

Upper respiratory tract infection

Following on from respiratory problems, the vet may decide that an upper respiratory tract infection is responsible for any breathing diffi-culties and may prescribe antibiotics and an anti-mucolytic like Bisolvon which will loosen any blockages.

Symptoms are very similar to our own 'common cold', with sniffling and a runny nose.

Vitamin deficiency

Vitamin deficiencies are not normally seen in wild animals, which usually subsist on a very balanced diet. They may, however, suffer during any prolonged spell in captivity. To avoid this always give a vitamin supplement to *all* wild animals.

Vomiting

Surprising though it may seem, I have not witnessed vomiting in wild mammals except in serious cases like poisoning, distemper and parvo-virus. All vomiting must be **referred to the vet** for assessment.

8

Skin Wounds, Abscesses, Fractures and Dislocations

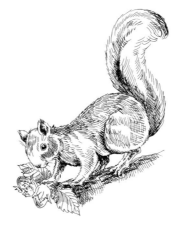

SKIN WOUNDS

The most noticeable difference between skin wounds in birds and mammals is that mammals are highly susceptible to infection in the wounds, whereas birds are reasonably resilient.

In addition, mammals seem to have far more pain receptors and must be treated with compassion and an awareness that any treatment of a wound, abscess or fracture is likely to be accompanied by pain for the patient. Most wild mammals will not yelp like a dog when they are hurt, they will bite or suffer in silence.

Most mammals will soldier on with a skin wound until infection finally slows them down enough to be spotted and then caught. These types of wounds can usually be attributed to bites or cut wounds from line or wire netting. Fresh wounds are usually the results of encounters with motor cars, lawn mowers, strimmers and dogs, where the victim is spotted immediately and taken to a care facility.

Fresh wounds will probably be bloody, whereas **infected wounds**

may not be obvious but need to be sought out. Look for signs such as matted fur over a wound site or a soft swelling, which sometimes shows pus but often just looks like an extension of the animal.

Before any attempt is made at treating a wound the animal must be assessed for its propensity to bite or kick (see Ch. 6, p. 116).

I WOULD NOT RECOMMEND THAT AN INEXPERIENCED PERSON EVEN ATTEMPTS TO HANDLE SOME OF THE MORE DANGEROUS ANIMALS UNLESS THE ANIMAL IS GENUINELY COMATOSE. EVEN THEN, A BANDAGE MUZZLE SHOULD BE TIED ON BEFORE ATTEMPTING CLOSE TREATMENT.

Species that I have in mind in this category are badgers, foxes, otters, seals, mink, martens and wild cats. Other smaller biting species which can be held in the heavily gloved hand include squirrels, weasels and stoats, edible dormice, water voles, large bats. Mammals which may bite but are not usually a hazard are hedgehogs, mice, small bats, smaller voles and shrews.

Rabbits and hares may kick out with their back legs, which should be controlled, but remember that rabbits, in particular, have weak backs.

Deer will also kick with their back legs or throw their heads about. Both actions can cause serious injury to a handler. Muntjac may use their antlers or sharp tusks to slash out at a handler.

The only 'sweetie' that shows no aggression is that now extremely rare common dormouse.

Finding and cleaning

Provided the casualty is under control, sedated or even anaesthetised, every wound should be clipped clear of hair or spines (see Ch. 7, p. 146). A wad of gauze in the wound whilst doing this will stop any falling in. The best tool for this job is a pair of curved scissors which make the accidental cutting of the skin unlikely. Electric dog clippers are used in veterinary practices for cutting back fur, but they are useless on hedgehog spines which have to be cut back with scissors.

The wounds should then be washed thoroughly with dilute Savlon or, preferably, dilute Hibiscrub (see Ch. 2, p. 47). A 10ml or 20ml syringe fitted with a blunt nozzle enables the dilute disinfectant to be flushed deep into the wounds and under the skin edges, removing every trace of debris. Regular wound cleaning can be further improved with the use of a 'Water Pik', a dental cleaning gadget imported from America and now sold in this country.

From then on, fresh clean wounds that do not need suturing will more than likely heal themselves. Healing can be accelerated by the application of Scherizorb gel (Smith & Nephew), available from any chemist. If the skin surrounding the wound moves over the underlying muscle layer, and if there is no infection, the exposed edges will benefit from being sutured together. Dirty or infected wounds should be cleaned with Dermisol Multi-cleanse Solution (Smith-Kline Beecham) and packed with Dermisol Cream to help remove stubborn dirt and necrotic (dead) tissue.

Enclosed wounds

Any enclosed wounds – ideal sites for anaerobic infection, where bacteria flourish without the need for air – could be flushed with metronidazole (Torgyl Solution – RMB) under the direction of a veterinary surgeon. There appear to be varying schools of thought as to whether a wound should be covered or left open to the air. I prefer the latter, although an open wound does need more regular attention, cleaning and medication. If the wound does need covering then a Melolin non-stick, absorbent dressing pad should be used.

Superficial wounds

Superficial infected wounds on the legs may need a long-term antiseptic application to clear away dirt and necrotic (dead) tissue. A povidone iodine non-adherent dressing (Inadine-Johnson & Johnson), available from chemists, will clean and help heal the wound.

In assessing the wound, imagine if you yourself had suffered a similar cut or graze. Would you want antibiotic cover from your doctor? If you think so, then take the animal to a vet, but if not, the preferable course, then let the wound heal on its own. But watch it for the first signs of infection or pus, when antibiotics may be the only answer.

SUTURING

Imagine yourself having stitches put in to close a wound. It hurts and will cause the same varying degrees of discomfort to any other mammal.

There is an alternative for small wounds and tears in a bat's wing and that is to use tissue glue (Vetbond – 3M), a super-glue that sets instantly as it touches the moisture of skin across a wound. However, if it will not hold the wound closed then suturing is the only answer.

ANY WOUND THAT WILL NOT CLOSE SHOULD BE REFERRED TO A SYMPATHETIC VET WHO CAN SUTURE IT UNDER LOCAL OR GENERAL ANAESTHETIC.

Incidentally, the practice of chilling bats in a refrigerator before suturing, or applying other treatment, is inhumane because although the bat may fall torpid it will still feel pain. Anaesthesia with Isoflurane is the only sound way to deal with bat injuries.

A new method of suturing skin tears in animals is the use of a staple suture, for example Elite Disposable Skin Stapler. It sounds very painful, but is very quick and effective, except perhaps in deer, as they have very tough skins. A special staple remover is needed to remove the sutures once the wound has healed.

INFECTED WOUNDS AND ANTIBIOTICS

We can automatically assume that any wound, other than a burn, is infected. Some fresh wounds can be cleaned and disinfected but in the main, wild mammals are not compromised until infection has taken over. The first noticeable sign of an infected wound is its smell, caused by the different bacteria attacking the exposed tissue.

After clipping and thoroughly cleaning the wound it can be further sanitised by irrigating it with dilute hydrogen peroxide. Bought at any chemist, the standard strength is '20vols'. Mixed with 95% water, the dilute hydrogen peroxide produced will, on contact with tissue, release oxygen, produce water and a foaming action that will disturb much of any residual matter in the wound.

A final flushing with clean water will leave a wound as clear as possible. With heavily infected wounds we have found that flushing with gentamicin, an antibiotic, acts against a broad spectrum of bacteria present in this type of wound.

Finally, packing the wound with amoxycillin or clindomycin powder hits practically all the bacteria resistant to gentamicin, prompting a rapid and successful healing. All these products are the domain of the veterinary surgeon who should be encouraged to try topical application of antibiotics to infected wounds.

Some bacteria are particularly resistant to many antibiotics and may need the use of a sensitivity test to establish a specific treatment to use. Many vets can provide this type of laboratory service by processing a sterile swab dipped in the infected material.

Many wounds, particularly those of hedgehogs, will only respond if given the appropriate antibiotics. As well as topical antibiotics, the vet should also institute a course of parenteral antibiotics by injection. The choice is his but antibiotic powders sprinkled on the animal's food have little or no effect on an infection and should be resisted even if the vet is persistent. Oral antibiotics do have a place in wildlife care but these are never in powder form – capsules or tablets that can be hidden in the food are better, particularly for those larger, harder-to-handle animals like badgers or foxes.

ORAL ANTIBIOTICS SHOULD NEVER BE GIVEN TO DEER, RABBITS OR HARES. These must receive injectable antibiotics followed up with pro-biotics to re-establish any gut flora destroyed by the antibiotics. Leo-Cud (Leo) is particularly useful to stimulate rumen activity in deer.

Infected wounds should be allowed to **heal from the inside out**. If the orifice closes over then any infection will be trapped inside, forming an abscess. Do not suture but keep infected wounds open and if necessary pull away any scabbing that might seal them. Regular cleaning and the application of Dermisol Multicleanse Solution or Ointment, once the infection is under control, will speed granulation, the cell building that is the process of healing.

I prefer to leave infected wounds uncovered, but if there is the danger of further contamination from food and other sources, the wound can be covered with a light dressing of Mclolin or Kaltostat (Hoechst), one of the new ion-active absorbent wound dressings. The latter should be cut and shaped to fit the orifice exactly. Melolin dressings should be changed every day and Kaltostat every three days.

ABSCESSES

Any unusual swelling (except on the stomach area) on a mammal should be suspected of being an **abscess**, a localised accumulation of pus

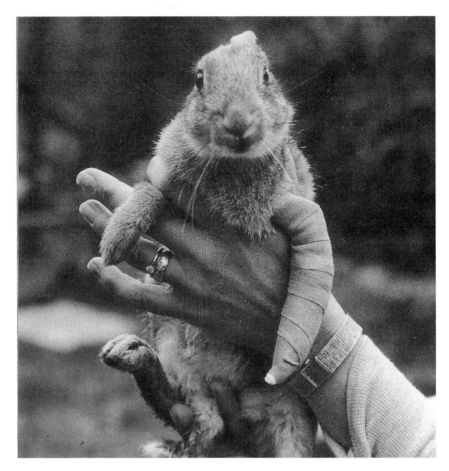

Never give rabbits oral antibiotics

surrounded by a fibrous capsule. It is painful and could be dangerous in spreading infection into the bloodstream and causing septicaemia. Clean off the area and if necessary clip away any hair or spines. If the swelling is on the abdomen it may be the result of a rupture so do no more than refer the animal to the vet.

Any other swelling should be rinsed with surgical spirit and a sterile hypodermic needle passed just through the skin to allow some of the contents out. As the needle is withdrawn some of the contents will seep out. This can be either blood, pus or fluid. If pus appears, then the hole should be enlarged by gently inserting the tip of a sterile pair of dressing scissors and opening them slightly.

By squeezing the swelling, all the infection can be expelled and washed away with dilute Savlon or Hibiscrub (see Ch. 2, p. 47). The abscess itself will then need flushing with a 10% solution of hydrogen peroxide followed by dilute Savlon or Hibiscrub. A final rinsing with metronidazole, available from a vet, will kill any remaining deep-seated anaerobic bacteria.

Much of the tissue and skin over the abscess will die off and can be picked clear with forceps. Like an infected wound, an abscess heals from the inside out so should be kept open and free of pus or necrotic (dead) tissue.

Some animals, notably rabbits, produce inspissated pus which is very thick and will need removing with forceps rather than by simply squeezing the abscess.

If there is any doubt about a swelling, or if pus does not seem to be present, then refer to the veterinary surgeon as the problem could be a tumour, haematoma or cellulitis (tissue inflammation).

FRACTURES

Fractures in mammals are extremely serious but can heal quite readily if given a chance and the appropriate treatment. They are generally the

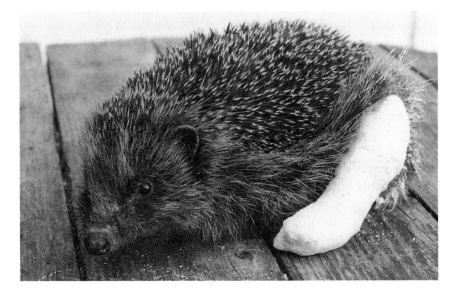

It is amazing how many hedgehogs suffer broken legs when they have never been near a road

result of collision or falling incidents, although it still remains a mystery as to how so many hedgehogs manage to break their legs when they have been nowhere near a road.

The first thing to remember with any fracture or suspected fracture that it is **extremely painful**, especially if the animal is moved. I recently came across a National Trust ranger who, on being called to a fallow deer knocked down by a car, promptly dragged it by its back legs into nearby undergrowth to shoot it. That deer possibly had one or more fractures so dragging it in this way could have grated broken bones together causing excruciating pain. I never agree with an animal being shot out of hand other than by a veterinary surgeon, who alone has the expertise to assess an animal's injuries and establish a prognosis. But if that deer *had* to be moved it should have been rolled onto a stretcher, plank of wood or blanket and carried off the road and kept still until expert help had been summoned.

Once again, imagine the animal casualty to be a human. Nobody would attempt to move a human road casualty until an ambulance had arrived in case any fractures were made worse, possibly causing fatal embolisms, haemorrhages or, at best, puncturing the overlying skin allowing infection to enter the fracture site.

I realise that this 'wait for the ambulance' policy is not practical with animal casualties but I would ask that each one is treated as the finest bone china and **moved as little as possible** without the benefit of a stretcher for a large deer, a blanket or sheet of board for a fox, or a cardboard box for squirrels, rabbits or hedgehogs.

While it is not possible to apply temporary splints to injuries in large casualties such as badgers, foxes and otters, the broken legs of a deer benefit from being temporarily splinted at the scene of the accident. Pieces of wood held with strips of cloth holding the legs approximately in a natural position will help ease the deer's discomfort and prevent any further injury if the animal has to be moved. Badgers, foxes and otters will probably bite if you try to fit even temporary splints at the accident scene.

All the mammals with fractures benefit from pain relief with buprenorphine (Temgesic – R&C), and every suspected fracture **must be seen by the veterinary surgeon**.

TYPES OF FRACTURE

Leg fractures

The most obvious fractures suffered by mammals are leg fractures, which usually result in the leg below the fracture site hanging limply. Any movement may produce crepitus, wherein the bone fragments may be felt grating on each other, causing pain, but crepitus is not always present.

Mammal leg bones

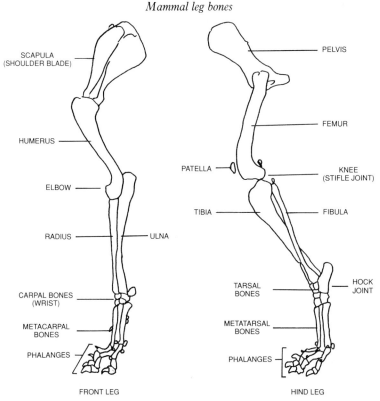

SCAPULA (SHOULDER BLADE)

HUMERUS

ELBOW

RADIUS — ULNA

CARPAL BONES (WRIST)

METACARPAL BONES

PHALANGES

FRONT LEG

PELVIS

FEMUR

PATELLA

KNEE (STIFLE JOINT)

TIBIA — FIBULA

TARSAL BONES

HOCK JOINT

METATARSAL BONES

PHALANGES

HIND LEG

Parts of the leg below the line of the chest and the abdomen that get broken are usually easily identified. In the front leg – equivalent to our own arms – are the radius and ulna, between the elbow and the wrist; and the metacarpal bones in the foot (our hand). The hind leg – equivalent to our shin bones – has the tibia and fibula between the knee (stifle joint) and ankle (hock joint) with the metatarsal bones in the foot.

Fractures in these bones can usually be treated with **immobilisation** in plaster or fibre-glass bandages, although the vet may wish to use metal fixings in some of the larger species. If the vet cannot be seen immediately then the fractured leg can be safely wrapped in a Robert Jones bandage: a heavily padded bandage that immobilises the fracture site but can still be easily removed and replaced with a more rigid cast. Any vet or veterinary nurse would be only too willing to demonstrate how to apply a Robert Jones bandage, an action which does stabilise a fracture and makes any further treatment that much more successful.

Above these relatively accessible fracture sites are the major leg bones: the humerus in the front leg and the femur in the hind leg. As most of these major bones are hidden in the body itself, it is not possible to stabilise them without stainless steel plates or intramedullary pins that fit inside the bone cavity. Most vets will carry out the operations but may be perplexed by the spines of a hedgehog. However, as the hedgehog's skin is so loose, the femur can, under anaesthetic, be slid from under the spiny rump, making the hedgehog the most simple of all femur pinning subjects.

Shoulder blades

The fracture of a shoulder blade can only be assessed with the help of an X-ray and should be suspected if any animal loses the use of its front leg without any obvious fractures of the long bones. Fractured shoulders are particularly damaging to animals like badgers, moles and hedgehogs, which need to dig to obtain their food.

Fractured pelvis

Similarly, fractures to the pelvis (hip bone) are best assessed under X-ray. Sometimes, if the animal is large enough, the veterinary surgeon may decide to operate but if not, then closely confined cage rest for at least six weeks may well see the animal recovered enough to be released.

During that period, however, there may well be a **disfunction of the bladder**, which should be emptied manually at least twice a day (see Ch. 7, pp. 146–7). If the animal is large and dangerous the vet may decide to insert a urinary catheter, which will allow the bladder to drain by gravity into an outside receptacle.

Extra attention should always be given to the prognosis for **female mammals with pelvic damage**. During labour, young have to pass through the pelvic bones and if there is any restriction the animal may not be able to give birth, resulting in death to both mother and babies. The female can be spayed but then there is the worry that the change in pheromones, the scents emitted during mating, may cause problems in its interactions with other wild members of its species. If there is any doubt about a female's ability to mate and give birth, it should not be released.

One other major problem occurring with **hip fractures** or **dislocations** is where the top of the femur refuses to sit in the hip joint, the acetabulum. The veterinary remedy, and it does work, is to remove the top of the femur (an excision arthroplasty), allowing a false joint to form, relieving the pain at the top of the femur resulting from grating on the pelvis. Animals which have received this operation usually improve enough to be released.

Fracture of the spine

The one horrific fracture that is the dread of anyone who works with animals is a fracture of the spine. And, contrary to some statements, hedgehogs can fracture their spine just like any other animal.

The typical symptoms of a broken back are **complete paralysis of the hind legs and tail**. Pinching the toes and tail, even with forceps, will produce no response; only an X-ray will show the extent of the damage. It could only be nerve damage that may in time respond, as will just a slight displacement of the vertebrae.

A severance or disruption of the spinal cord itself will never heal and the animal should be euthanased as the bladder will not function and all manner of other organs will fail eventually, killing the animal.

Damage to the nerves of the leg may well heal, although it does take a long time. Physiotherapy and electrical impulse treatment with an 'Activate' apparatus will speed healing. The one thing to watch for, as the legs recover their feeling, is the animal gnawing at its own feet, presumably as a response to the uncomfortable feeling of pins and needles as the nerves come back to life. As already suggested, the application of a bitter spray (Leo's Bitter Spray) or even encasing the leg in a mesh arrangement (such as ladies' hair curlers) may stop any further damage. Even an Elizabethan collar will help, if the animal leaves it on.

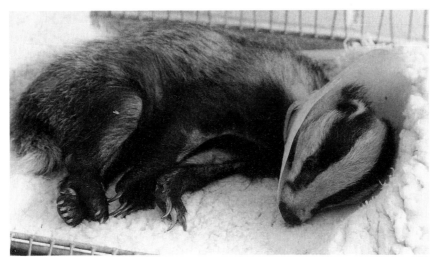

An 'Elizabethan collar' will prevent a badger from chewing at leg or foot injuries

Fractured skulls and noses

These are generally **left to heal on their own**, whereas fractures to the **lower jaw** can be **plated**, in the case of large animals, or **wired** in the smaller animals. A word of warning before plating lower jaws in deer: the vet should line up the teeth rather than the jawbone as is the normal practice in other mammals.

At the front of the lower jaw, where the two outer mandibles meet, is a cartilaginous joint known as the symphysis. This is often dislocated, allowing both mandibles to move independently. A sterile wire can be passed either over the incisors or through the jawbones to stabilise the juncture until it heals.

Fractured tails

Tails are very often fractured and generally the injury has no effect on the short-tailed animals like hedgehogs, rabbits and badgers. Animals that use their tails – squirrels, foxes, dormice and harvest mice – are lost without them, so every effort should be made to splint a broken tail with a strip of bamboo although it will probably not heal and have to be amputated, after which the casualty must be kept in captivity.

183

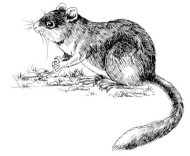

A dormouse needs its long tail, so any injury must heal perfectly

Bat wing fractures

Fractures in the minute bones of bat wings can be immobilised by simple adhesive plaster. Any tears over the bones can be sealed with tissue glue (Vetbond – 3M).

DISLOCATIONS

Dislocations occur where the end of one of the long bones or the lower jaw are wrenched out of their sockets, either by collision or trapping incidents. Like fractures, they are very painful to the mammal and should only be reduced under anaesthetic.

Some joints, particularly deer hip joints, are notoriously shallow, requiring the vet to introduce a toggle pin and a braided nylon round ligament prosthesis.

A dislocated bottom jaw can often be reduced under general anaesthesia by placing a length of 1–3cm diameter wooden rod across the mouth and sliding the joint back into position. The mouth may need taping closed (between meals) for some days afterwards.

ALL DISLOCATIONS SHOULD BE TREATED AS EARLY AS POSSIBLE OR ELSE THE BODY'S HEALING PROCESS TAKES OVER AND CONSTRICTS MUSCLES AND TENDONS, MAKING REDUCTION INCREASINGLY DIFFICULT. A TEMPORARY STRAPPING WILL PREVENT ANY FURTHER DAMAGE UNTIL A VET CAN INTERVENE.

AMPUTATIONS

Sometimes, with the best will in the world and plenty of care, the vet will have no alternative other than to amputate a leg or the tail. Various species cope with amputations in different ways, although they all benefit from extra fluid therapy after their operations.

No mammal should be allowed to struggle on if it has to lose two legs and even those that lose one leg and a tail should be closely monitored in case they cannot cope. I think it is inadvisable to release any animal that has lost a leg, although this does raise the question of euthanasia in particularly irascible and dangerous animals like adult deer. Most other species will settle to a life in captivity or even semi-captivity, where they can be helped if they get into trouble. For instance, any three-legged hedgehogs we treat are released into walled gardens, where they lead a subsidised natural life and do not have to cope with the hardships of a totally wild environment.

Our experience with different species shows the following:

rabbits and **hares** cannot cope with losing a back leg but can manage without a forelimb.

Squirrels cannot lose even one leg and without their tails cannot climb or balance.

Hedgehogs can manage on three legs.

Badgers manage on three legs but cannot dig without a front leg.

Foxes are as agile as ever on three legs but may suffer if they lose a tail as well.

Many **wild deer** manage on three legs but will meet trouble eventually.

A **young deer** soon learns to cope minus one leg but should never be released.

Most other mammals can cope with the loss of a limb, although I have no experience of a seal without a flipper or tail. Bats without part of a wing have been kept as molly-coddled pets by many people. They do, however, need constant attention and assistance in feeding.

Great strides are being made in human orthopaedic surgery with the use of bone glues, carbon-fibre rods and completely new thinking on casting and immobilisation. An apparently hopeless animal case may just be able to be solved by a human orthopaedist at the local hospital. It's worth a try if there seems to be no way with standard veterinary techniques. However, a veterinary surgeon *must* be in attendance during any surgery.

9

Housing, Feeding and Release

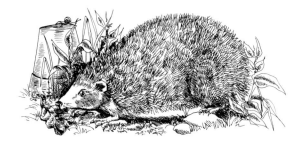

Housing

British mammal species vary so much in size that a mixture of containers or cages is necessary to cope with animals that may be either as small as a mouse or as large as a horse.

Any casualty will benefit at first from an added heat source **except for seals and adult deer**, animals that can easily suffer from hyperthermia, over-heating (see Ch. 7, pp. 155–6). These large animals will benefit from protection from adverse weather conditions but will need no further heat. In fact if, during the summer, they seem to be suffering from the warmth, some form of cooling of their quarters can be very helpful, but be careful of the draught created by a fan.

Draughts can cause all manner of problems even to animals that appear to be in a warm environment. Always try the old boy-scout wind-testing trick of wetting a forefinger just to see if a blast of cold air is whistling under the door or through a gap in a shed.

Apart from seals and deer, all other animal casualties should be taken into a warm environment. A house is suitable, but an outbuilding without auxiliary heat is going to be too cold.

There are various ways of providing **extra warmth**, the simplest being a hot water bottle wrapped in an old towel. However, as this needs changing regularly, a red light bulb suspended above the casualty will provide a certain amount of heat. British wild mammals are colour blind so will be unaware of the light given off by the red bulb.

There are on the market at pet stores, black lights especially designed for reptiles and small farm animals. Known as infra-red lamps or ceramic lamps they emit heat and no light, so are ideal for birds as well as mammals. Heated pads can be placed under a casualty's bedding but care must be taken that the animal is moved regularly and does not receive too much heat in one area of the body.

For the smaller animals, hospital cages designed for birds will provide a warm environment but, once again, care has to be taken and a comatose animal needs to be moved regularly from one spot to another.

BEDDING

Warm bedding that can be easily changed then discarded or washed will give any animal a sense of wellbeing as well as helping it recover. I would not, at the outset, recommend hay or straw, as the animal may hide itself, making it impossible to monitor its progress. Also, hay or straw will add to the dangers of contamination to any wounds; hay, in particular, may create a ligature around a part of any animal pacing or circling, a common habit with many wild mammal casualties.

For really small mammals like voles, mice or shrews, we provide **paper towels** as bedding. Bats are allowed to climb or hang on **cotton towels** fixed to the walls of their container. Any towels with shreds, holes or strands hanging should be discarded and never used for any animal in case they get caught, or choke trying to chew the threads.

Old hand or bath towels give good bedding to all the larger species, but use a **'Vet-bed'** for any casualty that cannot move. Vet-beds allow any urine to pass through, keeping the animal dry and free from urine-scalding or pressure sores.

Large deer are kept on **hay** purely because nothing else is suitable and they can eat their bedding to keep their stomachs active.

Seals require no bedding, just a clean, not too cold area to lie on. **'Warm' concrete** is available from builders' merchants and should be considered if seals are regularly taken into care.

HOLDING CAGES

These, of course, vary from animal to animal, but if I list the types of cage we use for various species it will give a lead to the requirements of any casualty. However, cardboard boxes, ice-cream tubs and other secure boxes will do if no sophisticated cage is to hand.

Mice, **voles** and **shrews** are kept in small plastic fish tanks with top-opening lids. The lids are perforated so overhead heat can be provided with one of the lamp-type heaters.

Bats are kept in specially made boxes after the design in the Nature Conservancy Council's (now English Nature) *Bat Workers' Manual*.

Squirrels, **weasels**, **stoats**, **small rabbits** and **hares** are kept initially in hospital cages and transferred to wooden cages when they are fitter.

Hedgehogs, **rabbits** and **hares** are placed in cages 1m × ½m × ½m with an overhead heat source at one end allowing the animal room to move away if it becomes too hot.

Badgers, **foxes**, **otters** and **mink** are kept in strong metal cages with vertical bars so they cannot lock their jaws onto the grilles. Heat for comatose animals is provided via radiant heaters.

Deer are kept to begin with in wooden boxes with wire mesh tops covered to prevent any outside vision. The boxes just allow the deer to stand but do not have any headroom, so the deer cannot jump and hurt itself. The wooden floor gives a good purchase for the hooves, which would slide on a metal base. The boxes are long enough and wide enough to allow the deer to walk around but not to damage itself.

RECOVERY CAGES

Once the animal's health has improved, it is put into an outside pen for acclimatisation before release. The important thing here is to prevent the patient escaping before you consider it ready, possibly into an unsuitable neighbourhood.

Mice and all the tiny mammals are kept in their plastic tanks throughout treatment, although some of them may chew through the plastic lids unless they are watched closely.

Bats are given exercise in a small mesh aviary, although a living room, with net curtains over the windows and all doors closed, could serve the purpose.

Weasels and **stoats** are kept in hutches with small mesh wire fronts and top-opening lids. These are portable enough to be taken directly into the field for releasing.

Squirrels can be kept in small mesh aviaries but notice should be taken of the law regarding their release (see Appendix III).

Rabbits and **hares** do well in standard rabbit hutches.

Hedgehogs can exercise in collapsible wire mesh pens like the Majestic Pens from Shaws Pet Foods of Aston Clinton, Buckinghamshire.

Badgers, **foxes** and **otters** will dig or climb their way out, so should be kept on concrete in a large pen made of heavy-duty welded wire with a wooden housing at one end.

Deer are better not moved once they have recovered, so are best allowed exercise in a small paddock from where they are to be released. Alternatively, they should be sedated before being caught up and taken to a place of release.

FEEDING

The nutritional requirements of mammals may not be as varied as those for birds but they are still just as important if the animal, when released, is to have the best chance of survival. It's crucial to know which animals require meat and which subsist on a vegetable diet; it's no good trying to change an animal's eating requirements – a carnivore will not be able to digest enough of a vegetarian diet and herbivores would never cope with a meat meal. To add to this, *nothing* will survive on bread and milk. Bread and milk is only a placebo, initiated by the Victorians, and is indigestible by British wildlife.

All food should have a vitamin supplement added. The simplest way is to use one of the multi-vitamin powders sprinkled on the bowl of food.

ORPHANS

Baby mammals of all species regularly need rearing. The feeding in most cases is simple – warm unpasteurised goat's milk. There are only a few exceptions: hedgehogs, rabbits and hares will benefit from the addition of goat's colostrum to their early feeds of goat's milk. Seals will thrive on a liquidised fish diet, delivered through a funnel and tube.

Adult diets

Mice, voles	Uncooked porridge oats, rabbit food, proprietary mouse diets, greenstuff, fruit.
Shrews	Pinkie maggots, mini-mealworms, insects.
Bats	Mealworms, pinkie maggots.
Moles	Mealworms, earthworms, cut-up mice*
Hedgehogs	Tinned dog or cat food (young on puppy food).
Squirrels	Peanuts, fruit, cuttle fish.
Dormice	Apples, peanuts.
Stoats, weasels	Mice or day-old chicks*
Foxes	Mice, chicks, rabbits* (young on puppy food).
Badgers	Rats, mice, chicks,* some peanuts and root vegetables (raw).
Otters, mink	Rats, mice, chicks,* some fish.
Deer	Coarse goat mix, browsing leaves.
Seals	Fish with a vitamin supplement.
Rabbits, hares	Rabbit mix plus grazing.

*Day-old chicks, mice, rats, rabbits are available frozen. They are essential for all the carnivores. Add a multi-vitamin supplement to all diets. Maggots and mealworms should have vitamins added the moment they arrive. Maggots are available at angling shops whereas the other diets suggested can be ordered from advertisements in the weekly paper *Cage and Aviary Birds*.

NON-RELEASABLE MAMMALS

Apart from the correct diet and as near-natural housing as possible, consideration should be given to the community spirit of a captive wild mammal. Many like to be alone, but others will pine away unless they have the company of their own species.

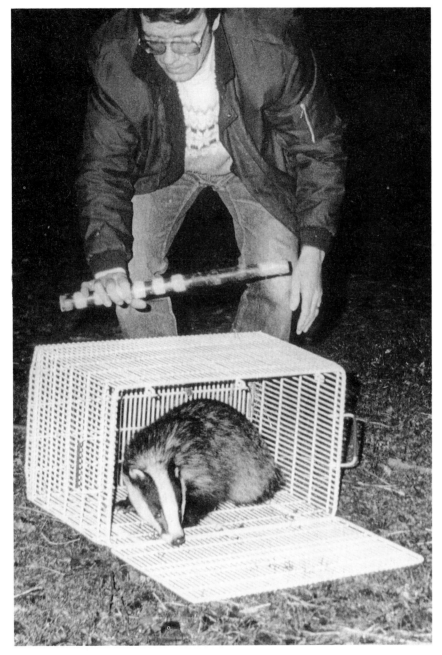

Always release badgers where they were found

My experience has been that **hedgehogs, muntjac,** some **squirrels, moles** and **shrews** like to be on their own. Although one pair of muntjac or a few females will thrive, two males will fight.

Similarly, although other deer may live together in harmony for most of the year, the males become aggressive during the rut. Neutering is a possible answer.

Badgers will usually mix, although an occasional aggressive animal may have to be kept on its own.

RELEASE

Much has been written about the suitability of a wild mammal for release. To my mind, if the animal is fit and there is an available food source, then it will cope. Look how the domestic cat fares in the wild and it has few of the wild instincts that truly wild animals possess.

It's not good enough, however, just to throw an animal out of your front door. Look at its lifestyle: will it find food? Will it be a nuisance to somebody? Are you releasing it into another's territory where it will have to fight for survival?

We have been releasing wild animals for fifteen years and have had no problems. We look at each species and give it the best chance and all the back up it needs, if necessary providing a feeding station until the animal itself decides not to come back.

These are some of our procedures for different species:

Mice, voles, shrews are released in good hedgerows where there is plenty of ground cover.

Bats are released where they were found although, at the moment, we are looking into the survival capabilities of bats with no known territory.

Moles are released in deciduous woodland – their preferred habitat.

Hedgehogs are released into known gardens where they have access to at least ten other gardens. A nest box and feeding station are provided initially.

Dormice are released, via a nest box and feeding station, into established dormouse habitat, usually in coppiced hazel wood.

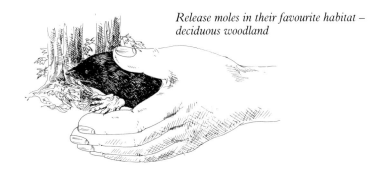

Release moles in their favourite habitat – deciduous woodland

Stoats and weasels thrive in traditional thick hedgerows.

Foxes are either released where they came from or into vacant fox territory on non-hunting ground and near to towns or villages where they can find a food source.

Badgers are released exactly where they were found or, if there is any doubt about their potential survival (mainly because of persecution by man), they are established in an empty or artificial sett.

Otters There are otter release programmes operating in Wales and Yorkshire. Any for release are better off introduced through this programme.

Deer Muntjac, roe and Chinese water deer are released individually into suitable woodland. Fallow and red are released where the species has a presence.

Seals When released off the coast where there are similar species, they will soon integrate with the wild population.

Rabbits and hares should only be released on meadow land with the full acceptance of the landowner.

In general, tame or imprinted animals should never be released. However, in saying that, I have known tame badgers and handleable hedgehogs to integrate with wild animals in a suitable, that is, safe area. But most tame animals will meet difficulties, not the least of them being that because they are not afraid of humans, they are vulnerable to persecution by them.

10

Reptiles and Amphibians

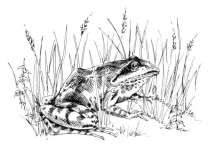

An example of the public's current increasingly favourable outlook on anything that is wild and natural is that people are less willing to kill a snake or dismiss a toad as a matter of course just because they are misunderstood creatures. As a consequence, more casualties are being brought to us, especially the toads that are injured while migrating across roads in spring and the frogs caught in the lawn mower.

Very little work has been carried out on the treatment of the British reptiles and amphibians, so any rehabilitation has to be an improvisation or adaptation of the procedures for exotic ectotherms (cold-blooded animals).

In short, any snake, lizard, frog, toad or newt taken into care probably has some form of traumatic injury. The first thing to remember is that **lizards** (and this includes slow worms) have the ability to discard their tails to confuse a predator. The tail will grow again with no intervention from humans, so the animal can be released if this is the only injury. **Newts** have the ability to regrow legs, so, once again, there is no need to intervene.

SNAKES

Other injuries will need some help. Firstly, snakes are very susceptible to dehydration so any casualty should be stomach-tubed with warmed

Hartmanns Solution for two days, then given Lectade for a further two before any solid food is offered.

All British reptiles and amphibians are **carnivorous** and would normally take live prey. However, it would be inhumane to offer a snake a live mouse in captivity, so a warmed dead mouse, of a natural colour, can be offered. It may take some time for the snake to catch on, but pulling the mouse along on a piece of string will eventually deceive it enough that it strikes.

All snakes require **water** for bathing and drinking, especially the grass snake, which also relishes the occasional fish to swallow. As with birds, fish-eating snakes require a vitamin B1 supplement to combat thiamine deficiency.

Any wounds that need suturing should be referred to a vet who specialises in reptiles. Sometimes a snake will be in trouble because it has been unable to shed its skin – a condition known as **dysecdysis**. The classic symptom is a clouding of the eye where the old skin has not come away. (Incidentally, snakes do not have eyelids, so they cannot close their eyes.) To assist a snake suffering with dysecdysis, place it between two wet towels held gently together to see if it can slough off the old skin on its own. If it does not manage it, then wiping the snake with damp cotton wool followed by dry cotton wool should clear the problem. Always wipe the cotton wool in the nose-to-tail direction. Never ever use tweezers or any rough abrasive to remove the old skin.

LIZARDS

Lizards can be treated in the same way as snakes, although their diet needs to be mealworms and small crickets. Slow worms, that look like snakes but can close their eyes like any true lizards, feed naturally on the small grey slugs found under stones and old planks of wood.

FROGS AND TOADS

These amphibians are very similar to each other, although the frog, with a liking for wet places such as long grass, has the ability to leap whereas the toad, which likes to live under rock, walks its way around the garden.

Many lose limbs in various accidents and whereas a toad can cope adequately without one back leg, a frog would be unable to survive. The loss of a front leg would only impair the ability of males of either species to carry out the amplexus grip used in mating.

Fractured legs can be splinted and, if the animal is kept in a warm environment of about 15°C, the break will eventually mend. Everything about amphibians takes a long time to heal, but a warm environment speeds the process up. Skin wounds can be sutured with fine vicryl, and keeping the casualty in shallow, very weak saline solution will keep the wound clean and again speed healing.

Fungus growths, especially on frogs, can be relieved by keeping the affected animal in fresh water, slightly coloured with potassium permanganate crystals.

We have recently come across an epidemic of a disease called 'red leg' in a population of free-living frogs. The disease manifests itself as red blotches on the frog's skin. Any healthy frogs found in contact with either live or dead specimens displaying these signs should be caught up and treated with antibiotics. Any interested vet will carry out a sensitivity test and prescribe a suitable remedy to be added to the frog's water.

Food for captive frogs and toads must be live. We have found waxworm larvae served in a dry aquarium to be readily taken by all our casualties.

There is still a great deal to be learnt about our native reptiles and amphibians and we at St Tiggywinkles are always willing to take on any casualty that needs attention or surgery.

EXOTIC SPECIES

With the advent a while back of ninja turtles, more and more exotic species of terrapin are being released or are escaping in the countryside. They are carnivorous and can wreak havoc on natural fish populations, as well as getting hooked occasionally by the fisherman.

The terrapins should be treated as aliens and not be re-released back into the wild but be handed over to one of the many exotic reptile collections at zoos or wildlife parks.

Similarly, tortoises are specialised exotic reptiles and should be given to one of the specialist tortoise sanctuaries now being set up.

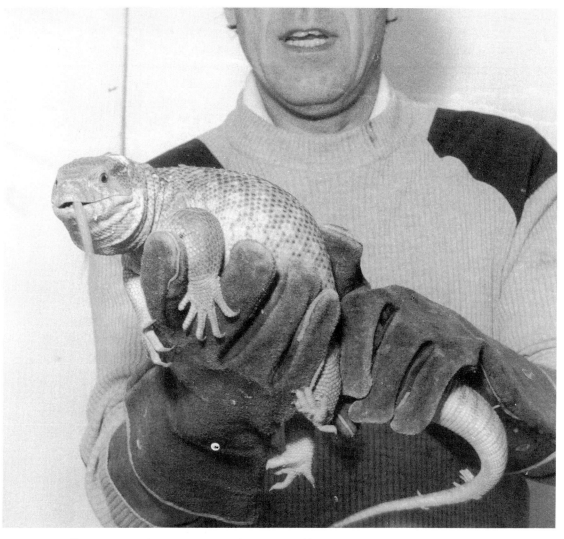

Return any exotic escapees to a reptile centre or wildlife park

Epilogue

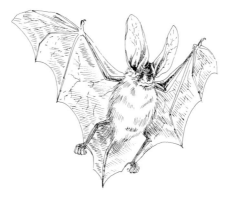

As more and more people become aware of the need to care for wildlife casualties, more and more previously unnoticed conditions are being found to perplex the rescuer and veterinarian alike. Similarly, as medicine and surgery progress, so more methods are found to cope with stubborn conditions. In the fifteen short years I have been dealing with sick or injured wild birds and other animals I have seen the advent of revolutionary new medicines and techniques, bringing hope and a cure where before there was nothing. And I am confident that new cures will be found for the new ailments.

Wildlife care is now the most important part of any conservation programme; the top of the conservation chain. No longer can it be ignored and now that we have opened the world's first Wildlife Teaching Hospital we are already seeing the benefit of sharing experiences with others who also care for wildlife casualties. The future of injured birds and animals is becoming more and more secure thanks to all those who willingly take waifs and strays into their own homes and care for them – you.

Further details and any help with a wildlife casualty can be obtained from: The Wildlife Hospital Trust, St Tiggywinkles, Church Farm, Aston Road, Haddenham, Aylesbury, Bucks HP17 8AF.

APPENDICES

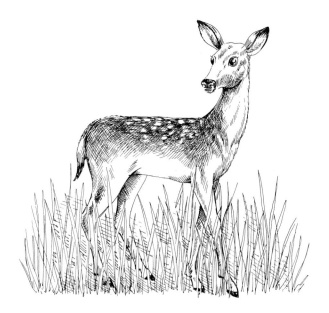

Appendix I

Drugs and dressings mentioned in the text

Available from most chemists
Canesten
Caustic pencil
Clearing fluid (10% potassium hydroxide solution)
Cod liver oil ointment
Complan
Daktarin oral gel
E45 cream
Ensure
Hibiscrub
Hydrogen peroxide solution 20vols
KY Jelly
Lacri-Lube eye ointment
Liquid paraffin
Melolin non-adhesive dressing
Non-adhesive cohesive bandage
Paraffin tulle
Potassium permanganate
Povidine iodine non-adherent dressing ('Inadine')
Savlon
Surgical spirit
Zinc oxide plaster

Available from vets under prescription
Amoxycillin
Antipamezole ('Antisedan')
Atropine sulphate
Aureomycin soluble powder

Bisolvon
Borgal
Chloramphenicol eye ointment
Chloromycetin succinate
Chloropromazine
Clindomycin capsules ('Antirobe')
Dexamethasone
Dextrose/saline (4% dextrose & 0.18% sodium chloride)
Dopram V drops
Finadyne injection for dogs
Frusemide ('Lasix')
Fulcin
GAC ear drops
Gentamicin
Griseofulvin
Haemaccel
Hartmanns solution
Hypromellose eye drops
Isoflurane – needs oxygen
Kaobiotic tablets
Medazolam ('Antisedan')
Metronidazole ('Torgyl Solution')
Myllophyline V
Nizoral
Oterna ear drops
Oxytocin
Panalog ointment
Parentrovite
Pipothiazine palmitate ('Piportil-Depot')
Temgesic
Ventipulmin
Vetibenzamine

Vitamin B12 injection
Vitamin K injection

Available from vets without prescription
Can-addase enzyme supplement
Dermisol multi-cleanse solution
Fungassay test kit
Geeling giving set
Hypodermic needles
Ivermectin ('Ivomec')
Kaltostat veterinary
Kaosal
Lectade
Leo-Cud
Liquivite
Scalpel blades
Spartrix
Spray-on plastic skin ('Op-site')
Syringes
Tissue glue ('Vetbond')
Vitamin powder ('Vit-a-min+zinc')

Available from other sources
Battle fly and maggot paste – agricultural merchants
Parvocide – agricultural merchants
Prosecto dried insect food – Haiths, Park St., Cleethorpes, South Humberside DN35 7NF
Rid-mite powder – pet stores
Sluis Universal Food – pet stores
Sterile bone meal – pet stores
Swarfega – agricultural merchants

Appendix II

Equipment mentioned in text and suppliers

From vets or medical suppliers
Artery forceps
Aurioscope
Curved scissors
Electric heat pads
Needle holders or Gillies
Plastic leg-splints
Spreulls needles
Stethoscope
Suture materials

From pet stores
Budgerigar water fountain
Ceramic heat lamps
Kitten & puppy feeders
Majestic pens
Plastic pill-giver
Teats
Vet-bed

Advertised in Cage and Aviary Birds, *available from your newsagent*
Bird-catching nets
Frozen mice or chicks
Hospital cages
Live foods – mealworms etc.
Welded mesh

From MD Components, 211–13 High Town Road, Luton, Beds
Baskets
Crush cages
Fox cage trap
Grasper (dog catcher)
Pigeon trap
Stretchers
Thick gloves

From Thermocare Inc., 3004 Mission St., Santa Cruz, CA, USA
Nebulisers

From Shepherds Basket Works, Paigle Road, Aylestone, Leicester LE2 8PD
Columbo-clip and other pigeon-care equipment

From Southern Veterinary Services, Brooks Road, Lewes, E. Sussex BN7 2AL
'Water Pik'

From Canac Pet Products, Becks Mill, Westbury Leigh, Westbury, Wilts
Tick remover

Hardware stores
Fencing pliers

In view of the difficulty experienced in obtaining some of this equipment, St Tiggywinkles now has a small mail order department dealing with rehabilitation supplies. Please contact the Hospital direct for more information.

Appendix III

Some legislation affecting the care of wildlife casualties

Protection of Animals Act 1911, Protection of Animals
   (Scotland) Act 1912 and other amending legislation
   collectively 1911–88
Destructive Imported Animals Act 1932
Abandonment of Animals Act 1960
Deer Act 1963
The Veterinary Surgeons Act 1966

The Veterinary Surgeons Act 1966 (Schedule 3
   Amendment) Order 1991
Firearms Act 1968
Conservation of Seals Act 1970
Badgers Act 1973
Transit of Animals (General) Order 1973
Dangerous Wild Animals Act 1976
Wildlife and Countryside Act 1981

Appendix IV

Some useful addresses

British Waterways Board, Melbury House, Melbury
   Terrace, London NW1 6JX
Cats Protection League, 17 Kings Road, Horsham, West
   Sussex RH13 5PP
Department of the Environment, Tollgate House,
   Houlton Street, Bristol BS2 9DJ
English Nature (formerly Nature Conservancy Council),
   Northminster House, Peterborough, Cambs PE1 1UA
Forestry Commission, 23 Corstorphine Road, Edinburgh
   EH12 7AT
Henry Doubleday Research Association, National Centre
   for Organic Gardening, Ryton-on-Dunsmore, Coventry
   CV8 3LG
Hunt Saboteurs Association, PO Box 87, Exeter, Devon
   EX4 3TX
Institute of Terrestial Ecology, Monks Wood, Abbots
   Ripton, Huntingdon, Cambs PE17 2LS
League Against Cruel Sports, Sparling House, 83–87
   Union Street, London SE1 1SG
Lynx, PO Box 509, Dunmow, Essex CM6 1UN
Ministry of Agriculture, Fisheries and Food, Whitehall
   Place, London SW1A 2HH

National Federation of Badger Groups, 16 Ashdown
   Gardens, Saunderstead, South Croydon, Surrey CR2 9DR
National Rivers Authority, 30–34 Albert Embankment,
   London SE1 7TL
New Forest Deer Protection Council, Sims Cottage,
   Wilverley Road, Wootton, New Milton, Hants
   BH25 5TX
Royal College of Veterinary Surgeons, 32 Belgrave
   Square, London SW1X 8QP
Royal Society for the Prevention of Cruelty to Animals,
   Causeway, Horsham, West Sussex RH1 2HG
Royal Society for the Protection of Birds, The Lodge,
   Sandy, Beds SG19 2DL
Scottish Society for the Prevention of Cruelty to Animals,
   19 Melville Street, Edinburgh EH3 7PL
Sea Mammal Research Unit, British Antarctic Survey,
   High Cross, Madingley Road, Cambridge CB3 0ET
Soil Association, 86 Colston Street, Bristol BS1 5BB
Ulster Society for Prevention of Cruelty to Animals,
   11 Drumview Road, Lisburn, Co. Antrim BT21 7YF
Wildlife Hospital Trust, St Tiggywinkles, Church Farm,
   Aston Road, Haddenham, Aylesbury, Bucks
   HP17 8AF

Bibliography

BEYNON, P. H. and COOPER, J. E. (eds), *Manual of Exotic Pets*, BSAVA, 1991

BRINKER, W. O., PIERMATTEI, D. L. and FLO, G. L., *Handbook of Small Animal Orthopedics and Fracture Treatment*, Saunders, 1983

COLES, B. H., *Avian Medicine and Surgery*, Blackwell Scientific, 1985

COOPER, J. E., *Veterinary Aspects of Captive Birds of Prey*, Standfast, 1978

——, and ELEY, J. T., *First Aid and Care of Wild Birds*, David and Charles, 1983

CORBET, G. B. and HARRIS, S., *The Handbook of British Mammals* (third edn), Blackwell, 1991

CRAMP, S., *Handbook of the Birds of Europe, the Middle East and North Africa*, Oxford University Press, 1977

HICKMAN, M. and GUY, M., *Care of the Wild Feathered and Furry*, Unity Press, 1973

KING, A. S. and McLELLAND, J., *Birds, Their Structure and Function*, Baillier Tindall, 1984

LANE, D. R., *Jones's Animal Nursing*, Pergamon Press, 1989

McKEEVER, K., *Care and Rehabilitation of Injured Owls*, W. F. Rannie, 1979

MITCHELL-JONES, A. J., *The Bat Worker's Manual*, Nature Conservancy Council, 1987

RUDGE, A. J. B., *The Capture and Handling of Deer*, Nature Conservancy Council, 1984

SANDYS-WINSH, G., *Animal Law*, Shaw and Shaw, 1984

STOCKER, L., *The Complete Hedgehog*, Chatto & Windus, 1987

——, *The Complete Garden Bird*, Chatto & Windus, 1991

——, *Code of Practice*, Wildlife Hospital Trust, 1991

—— and KILSHAW, R., *Medications for Use in the Treatment of Hedgehogs*, Wildlife Hospital Trust, 1987

Tri-State Bird Rescue and Research Inc., *Oiled Bird Rehabilitation*, 1990

WHITE, J., *Basic Wildlife Rehabilitation*, Skills Seminar, International Rehabilitation Council, 1988

Index

Acknowledgements

My life seems to revolve round talk of injured animals and birds, with everyone I meet having to suffer my obsession. But many of these people have helped me learn the intricacies of running a hospital and gather the experiences for this book.

Our new hospital is now up and running. I believe due, in the main, to the efforts of my family, Sue, Colin and Andrea, and all my great team of volunteers who struggled on in Aylesbury, helped us move to Haddenham and now make the new premises flourish.

My two vets, John Lewis and Malcolm Paul, listen to my vagaries and have suggested many sophisticated innovations that have brought the joy of higher success rates. This, together with the support of our many sponsors, has given us the wherewithal, and a new hospital, to cope with the often desperate and horrifying things that happen to wildlife.

I appreciate the input of everybody who supports St Tiggywinkles, especially our members, who have made it such a driving force in the care of sick and injured wildlife. Thank you all, and thank you once again to Catherine Miller, the glutton for punishment who turns my manuscripts into legible print, even though I refuse to use a word processor.